Evidence-Based Practice in Athletic Training

Evidence-Based Practice in Athletic Training

Scot Raab, PhD, AT, LAT
Northern Arizona University

Debbie I. Craig, PhD, AT, LAT
Northern Arizona University

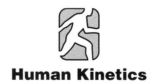

Human Kinetics

Library of Congress Cataloging-in-Publication Data

Raab, Scot, 1971- , author.
  Evidence-based practice in athletic training / Scot Raab, Debbie I. Craig.
    p. ; cm.
  Includes bibliographical references and index.
  I. Craig, Debbie I., author. II. Title.
  [DNLM: 1. Athletic Performance. 2. Evidence-Based Practice--methods. 3. Research Design.
QT 260]
  GV711.5
  613.7'11--dc23
                                    2015016723

ISBN: 978-1-4504-9815-9 (print)

The web addresses cited in this text were current as of August 2015, unless otherwise noted.

Acquisitions Editor: Joshua J. Stone; **Developmental and Managing Editor:** Amanda S. Ewing; **Copyeditor:** Patsy Fortney; **Proofreader:** Jan Feeney; **Indexer:** Nan Badgett; **Permissions Manager:** Dalene Reeder; **Graphic Designer:** Kathleen Boudreau-Fuoss; **Cover Designer:** Keith Blomberg; **Photo Asset Manager:** Laura Fitch; **Photo Production Manager:** Jason Allen; **Art Manager:** Kelly Hendren; **Associate Art Manager:** Alan L. Wilborn; **Illustrations:** © Human Kinetics, unless otherwise noted; **Printer:** Sheridan Books

Printed in the United States of America   10   9   8   7   6   5   4   3   2   1

The paper in this book is certified under a sustainable forestry program.

Human Kinetics
Web site: www.HumanKinetics.com

United States: Human Kinetics
P.O. Box 5076
Champaign, IL 61825-5076
800-747-4457
e-mail: humank@hkusa.com

Canada: Human Kinetics
475 Devonshire Road Unit 100
Windsor, ON N8Y 2L5
800-465-7301 (in Canada only)
e-mail: info@hkcanada.com

Europe: Human Kinetics
107 Bradford Road
Stanningley
Leeds LS28 6AT, United Kingdom
+44 (0) 113 255 5665
e-mail: hk@hkeurope.com

Australia: Human Kinetics
57A Price Avenue
Lower Mitcham, South Australia 5062
08 8372 0999
e-mail: info@hkaustralia.com

New Zealand: Human Kinetics
P.O. Box 80
Mitcham Shopping Centre, South Australia 5062
0800 222 062
e-mail: info@hknewzealand.com

We dedicate this work to our families.
Without their support,
we never would have completed
the many facets of this project!

Thanks to Amy, Jillian, Amelia, and to Isabella.

We love you!

Contents

Preface xi ▪ Acknowledgments xiii

Preface

Welcome to *Evidence-Based Practice in Athletic Training*. We're excited to offer this text to athletic trainers and other health care professionals as well as to students. As we reviewed resources to address the new requirements for athletic trainers' continuing education throughout the United States, we realized that a gap existed in the literature. We found no specific resource for learning how to use evidence-based practice (EBP) efficiently in the athletic training domain. Athletic training education programs currently teach EBP, along with basic research methods, but without a text devoted to or centered on topics specific to athletic training. Thus, this text serves two groups of people—certified athletic trainers and other health care professionals who seek to expand their knowledge and understanding of EBP, and athletic training students who are completing course work requiring an understanding of EBP and basic research methods in athletic training.

For students, this text provides a thorough knowledge and skill base in two areas: EBP and research design methods. Depending on the level of study, some students are required to design and complete research projects. Other students are required to evaluate research studies (evidence) through critical appraisal in many institutional settings. It is our hope that all athletic training students will be required to research, evaluate, and apply evidence-based practices and then critically appraise their own clinical practice using EBP methods. This text provides knowledge and easy-to-follow examples in each of these areas so that clinical practitioners can thrive in an EBP workplace and improve the health of their athletes.

For credentialed health care professionals who seek further knowledge and continuing education units (CEUs), this text provides an easy-to-follow description of EBP basic searching skills as well as exercises to help in applying those skills to the evaluation and application of the evidence related to their practice. For certified athletic trainers, the Board of Certification (BOC) currently requires 10 CEUs in EBP per two-year reporting period. This text and the accompanying electronic CEU quizzes meet the 10 CEU requirement, once successfully completed.

Organization

The text is organized in three parts: EBP basic searching skills, the evaluation and application of EBP, and general research methods in athletic training. Part I includes chapters on EBP models, including introductions to the levels of evidence and the five steps of searching for evidence, PICO question development and search techniques, and the advantages and disadvantages of research designs. These chapters give you the background necessary for implementing EBP in your daily athletic training practice.

Part II provides greater detail to help you determine the quality and utility of the research articles you find in your EBP searches. Chapters 4 through 6 describe diagnostic research, prognostic research, and systematic reviews and meta-analyses, respectively. Each chapter defines the research type, provides resources to help you find studies of that type, and describes how to critically appraise the studies you find. Chapters 7 and 8 provide overviews of clinical practice guidelines and the types of outcome measures used in EBP research, respectively. These two chapters provide further knowledge about how to appraise and use the results or outcomes of the studies you locate.

Part III addresses research methods and ethical research practice. Chapter 9 discusses the components of quantitative research and includes a brief review of statistical measures often used in athletic training research. Chapter 10 describes qualitative research methods, addressing the types of qualitative studies, how data are analyzed, and how to assess the trustworthiness, or validity, of these types of studies. Finally, chapter 11 reviews research ethics, including institutional review board policies and purposes, the six ethical principles of research, and why ethical research is critical.

You can approach any of these three areas independently or all three in succession, depending on your needs and prior knowledge. If you are a student or practitioner new to EBP, work your way through the entire text as presented. It is written concisely, and concepts are presented clearly and with ample athletic training examples. If you are a certified health care provider, you can use sections of the text for a home study program to earn CEUs to meet the BOC requirement of knowledge in EBP.

Following the presentation of concepts related to understanding or applying EBP principles are clinically based scenarios that you can use to apply your new knowledge to real-life situations. This will foster a deeper appreciation of the topic. Learning new concepts is fairly common for health care professionals; however, becoming proficient at applying EBP and research concepts is a more complex task that requires the performance of repeated exercises designed to promote learning. We hope you will take advantage of the clinically based scenario exercises throughout the text.

Instructor Ancillaries

For instructors of EBP courses, the following ancillaries are included:

- **Presentation package plus image bank:** More than 200 PowerPoint slides present the key concepts of every chapter. You can modify these slides to best fit your classroom discussions. In addition, an image bank of all the figures and tables is provided. These items can be added to the PowerPoint slides, used to create student handouts, and so on.

- **Instructor guide:** The instructor guide includes a sample syllabus and chapter-specific files with the chapter objectives, summary, individual student assignment suggestions, lab activity suggestions, class project suggestions, and annotated lists of additional readings.

The ancillaries can be accessed at www.HumanKinetics.com/EvidenceBasedPracticeInAthleticTraining.

We hope you enjoy learning with our text and materials as much as we've enjoyed creating them for you.

Acknowledgments

At times we come across books used in the realm of education that inspire and shape lives. Then, all too often, those books become dated, and updated editions fail to appear. However, having been through the writing of this text, we can now acknowledge the private, personal cost of publication. From time away from family and friends while working long hours in an office or dimly lit room illuminated only by a laptop so our loved ones could sleep, to the numerous missed meals and cold dinners suffering from what Scot's kids call love bites (small bites they take out before gently wrapping them in plastic and placing them in the fridge), authoring a text requires effort from others besides simply the authors. With that said, we'd like to acknowledge the team effort, especially of our families, with whom we are blessed to share this life.

PART I

Introduction

Part I presents basic knowledge of evidence-based practice (EBP), explains how to find the evidence, and describes general concepts used to evaluate research outcomes. Given the preponderance of evidence (i.e., research studies) available in the health care field, clinicians need a good grasp of these basics.

Chapter 1 presents many core concepts in EBC, including models of EBP, levels of evidence, the five steps of practicing EBP as a clinician, and applications to use when implementing EBP in your daily practices. Pay close attention to the levels of evidence discussion, because we do not go into further depth at other points in the text, and it is a critical concept to ground your understanding of the types of evidence you will find.

Chapter 2 uses some active learning. You will be asked to create a searchable question using the PICO technique and then to use that question through the rest of a five-step process to come up with an answer to your clinical question. The chapter also explains how to perform online searches efficiently and effectively. By the end of the chapter, you will already have your first EBP search completed and will be able to implement new evidence in your clinical practice.

Chapter 3 provides the basic knowledge necessary for understanding some of the statistical language you will encounter when reading and appraising research studies. Concepts you will learn include validity, reliability, sensitivity, and specificity. The chapter not only defines these important concepts but also provides examples in the field of athletic training to further your understanding.

After studying the three chapters in part I, you will be ready to learn about the types of evidence you will come across and how to appraise each type in part II.

CHAPTER 1

Evidence-Based Practice Models

Objectives

After reading this chapter, you will be able to do the following:

- Define evidence-based practice (EBP) and understand its importance to athletic trainers.
- Apply the five steps of keeping EBP athlete focused.
- Understand the levels of hierarchy of clinical research.

Athletic trainers (ATs), both students and professionals, often question the links among what they learn in didactic classroom settings, what they read in the athletic training literature, and what is practiced and observed in clinical settings. A person could state that this autonomy of practice and interpretation of application constitutes the art of athletic training. Often, a clear link exists between theory and practice; other times, the nuances of variations in courses of treatment are confounding. However, failing to incorporate new theories or evidence into practice because you are comfortable with the tried-and-true art of athletic training can compromise athlete care. To use your own time and that of your athletes wisely, and to effectively treat the presented conditions, you need to critically review all the information available, including new research, and arrive at logical conclusions.

Definition of Evidence-Based Practice

Evidence-based practice (EBP) is a systematic method of reviewing the best evidence, combining it with the art of athletic training or your clinical expertise, and making informed choices to treat the athlete.[1] Integrating EBP requires that you incorporate your clinical expertise, your athletes' values, and the best available clinical research into your practice. At its core, EBP is about focusing on athlete and clinical outcomes.

Clinical expertise is the culmination of your experience treating and providing care to athletes. It includes your personal values, preferences, experiences, and wisdom.[2] Clinical expertise develops from hours of observation and trial and error and can result in a sense of pride and emotion. An AT who is vested in caring for an athlete can be uncomfortable being wrong about an assessment or a rehab and treatment program. Likewise, facing a challenging clinical case, deciding on a course of action, and having that action confirmed by other health care providers can be very rewarding. This is the reason many ATs are wary of incorporating new techniques that are unfamiliar to them. However, such a guarded approach can keep them from remembering that optimal athlete outcomes are the most important goal.

Patient values are the preconceived ideas and beliefs each athlete brings to the clinical setting. Athletes all have their own distinctive concerns that you must address.[1] Often, the athlete arrives with a set feeling of trust in or distrust of ATs that has been cultivated from prior experience or social discussions. Furthermore, the athlete's values can be skewed by the appearance or functional use of the athletic training room and the amount of traffic. Some arrive lacking a clear understanding of the body and the healing process and may have set unrealistic time lines for their return to participation. This will influence their adherence to, or desire to complete, therapy. Treatment can be further confounded by comorbidities and the athlete's support network.[2] Although the challenge is unique for each athlete, as an EBP clinician, you must consider all athletes' perspectives.

Clinical research is a scientific and systematic process that generates evidence through hypothesis testing and sound methodology.[1,2] This is perhaps the most challenging portion of the EBP concept to incorporate. You may have limited experience analyzing peer-reviewed literature, and learning this process may thus appear daunting. Published studies should at a bare minimum introduce a research question, describe the methods used to assess subjects, outline the variables of interest, and explain the participant inclusion and exclusion criteria. The statistical analysis should align with the methods, and the authors should report only facts in the results section. The discussion or impression of the outcomes belongs in the conclusion or discussion section of an article. When assessing the quality of a clinical research article, ask the following questions:[3]

- Were eligibility criteria specified?
- Were subjects randomly assigned to groups, and was assignment concealed, if appropriate?
- Were subjects similar at baseline?
- As appropriate, were subjects, clinicians, and assessors blinded to the treatment of participants?
- Was the completion rate of participants 85% or higher?

Eligibility criteria are a set of delimiters that detail who can be included in a study. These might include age limits, an association with a specific sport, a particular injury or medical condition, ethnicity, or sex. You need to know whether the study will be relevant to the athlete in your care.

Randomization is important in research because it helps to determine whether something truly made an impact, or whether it might have occurred by chance alone or as a result of a preconceived bias. An unethical researcher might place participants in a study group according to a notion that one group will respond more favorably to the treatment, with the purpose of showing support for that treatment. Likewise, whether participants were blinded (not aware that they were placed in a control or experimental group) is an important consideration when reviewing a study. To help the researcher or support a product or treatment they favor, participants who are not blinded may alter their efforts on tests or skew their reporting.

The similarity of participants is also crucial when determining a study's relevance. Participants should be similar in such factors as age, sport, and condition. It would be inappropriate to conclude that a new treatment works if those in the experimental group receiving the treatment were vastly different from those in the control group who did not receive a treatment. Furthermore, blinding the assessors to the participants' treatment limits the possibility of assessor bias.

A study that uses a goniometer to assess the effects of two treatments on range of motion (ROM) is a good example of potential assessor bias. An assessor who believes that moist hot packs are more effective at increasing ROM than diathermy (electrically induced heat) might report higher ranges of motion posttreatment for participants receiving the moist hot packs. Again, blinding both subjects and assessors, as appropriate, and having similar subjects are all methods to increase trust in the outcomes.

Finally, researchers should report the participant completion rate to reveal the percentage of participants who dropped out of the study. A completion rate of less than 85% raises suspicion. Reviewers should question why so many participants dropped out. Was the study poorly organized? Was it painful? Was it too cumbersome or difficult?

With all of these aspects of research to consider, always keep the three components of EBP (clinical expertise, patient values, and clinical research) in mind. The bottom line is that EBP should always revolve around the athlete.[1]

Five Steps of Evidence-Based Practice

To use evidence-based practice and retain an athlete focus, follow these five steps:[2]

1. Create a clinically relevant and searchable question concerning your athlete.
2. Conduct a database search to find the best evidence.
3. Critically appraise the articles or evidence for quality.
4. Critically synthesize the evidence to choose and implement a treatment.
5. Assess the outcomes by monitoring the athlete.

Let's take a closer look at each of these steps.

• **Step 1:** The first step is to start with the athlete, establish the clinical concern, and build a clinical question that centers on solving the issue or treating the condition. Further details on developing a clinical research question are presented in chapter 2. In the meantime, remember that the clinical question should be focused and searchable. A question that is too narrow in scope will return limited results. One that is too wide will return excessive information, limiting your ability to incorporate the content into a treatment plan. For example, if you are curious about the ability of ultrasound to facilitate increased tissue extensibility and are treating an athlete with ITB syndrome, searching for *treat ITB with ultrasound* may result in few or no results. It is too narrow and specific. If you search for *ultrasound treatment,* the results will most likely be too wide. A more appropriate approach might be to search for *ultrasound AND connective tissue.* This would return studies related to ultrasound and its effects on connective tissue. This will not be specific to ITB, but because ITB involves connective tissue, the treatment parameters and outcomes may be similar enough to draw upon for clinical use.

• **Step 2:** This step pertains to conducting the database search and looking for the best evidence related to the athlete's condition or injury. Chapter 2 explains how to conduct the search (including Boolean modifiers and search engines and databases), format the question, and conduct the first search. With practice, you will become adept at completing this in minimal time.

• **Step 3:** Appraise the articles for quality and for whether they are applicable to your athlete.[1] Chapters 3 through 6 will help you learn how to do this. It is helpful to rate the quality and applicability of the studies you find on these two scales. A study may be of high quality but not applicable to your current athlete. For example, consider the effect of counterirritants. A research project that applied counterirritants to athletes with arthritis and found no improvement in range of motion at the fingers would not apply to an athlete's use of counterirritants to treat muscle spasms of the gastrocnemius. In this example, the study might be well designed but have no relevance to an athlete with a tight gastrocnemius. Conversely, a study of the effect of counterirritants on athletes with muscle spasms might be very applicable. However, if the article fails to report subjects' baseline measures, the inclusion or exclusion criteria, or the type of counterirritant used, this would indicate low quality. Without a certain amount of requisite data presented in the study, it would be impossible to devise a treatment plan.

• **Step 4:** This step involves critical processing and synthesizing. Integrating the evidence, your own clinical expertise and comfort in performing certain skills, and the values of the athlete will form the framework for your treatment plan.

• **Step 5:** This step returns to the athlete. You need to evaluate critically the progress and outcomes, reflecting on steps 1 through 4 and continually aiming to improve outcomes.

Levels of Evidence

Step 3 of the EBP process is appraising the research. Although this step is addressed throughout the textbook with various exercises, it is important to note here the levels of research evidence (figure 1.1).

From the bottom of the pyramid toward the top, the quantity of research diminishes but the relevance to clinical settings and the quality of the research increase. Background information and expert opinion are important but often lack strength when reviewed for the research controls noted earlier. Case reports and case series are not experiments; they are ex post facto reports on actual clinical events. They often present novel events that generate further hypotheses and lead to future research. They have value but are deficient in statistical validity because they lack control groups and sound experimental designs. An example of an important use of case series and reports is the recent increase in back-to-back Tommy John surgeries in professional baseball (i.e., a pitcher has a second failure of the ulnar collateral

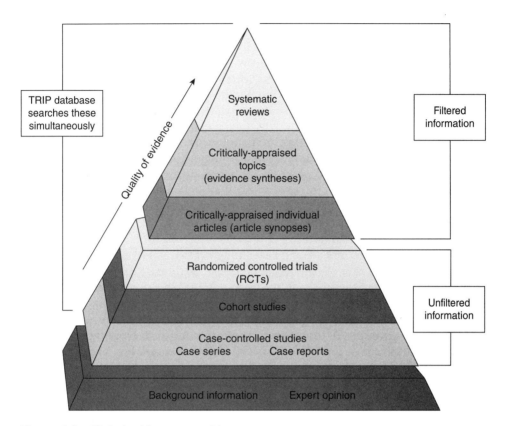

Figure 1.1 Clinical evidence pyramid.

ligament in the pitching arm and requires a second surgery). This raises the questions of surgical failure, insufficient rehabilitation, improper throwing mechanics, and the high velocity pitchers must maintain. At any rate, this archival data will result in future controlled studies.

Case control studies and cohort studies are similar in the questions they ask. However, case control studies look for the cause of a condition that has already occurred; it is a retrospective review of events. Cohort studies gather data prospectively on potential candidates of an injury, or those theorized to be at risk for injuries.[2] To help you understand these differences, let's consider a sprain to the anterior talofibular ligament. We want to look at a group of athletes with this injury and those without the injury who are similar in other factors (age, activity, sex). Looking backward, we are trying to assess what was different between the groups that may have contributed to the injury. This should lead to a potential intervention or future studies with greater experimental controls. This is an example of a case control study.

In a cohort study, we follow athletes going forward. Let's look at the example of replacing grass fields with turf. No injury has occurred at the present time, but going forward we will watch athletes playing on turf and athletes playing on natural grass to see whether certain injuries occur at different rates. If over a period of time we find a significant difference in the number of specific injuries, we might devise an intervention to decrease injury rates.

As we approach the top of the evidence pyramid, we find four of the highest-quality research types: **randomized controlled trials (RCTs), critically appraised topics (CATs), systematic reviews (SRs),** and **meta-analyses (MAs)**. An RCT starts with a similar group of participants representative of a population of interest. In athletic training, these are often athletes or physically active people. Participants are randomly assigned to either a control group receiving no treatment (or a sham group receiving a placebo) or an experimental group that is treated with an intervention the researcher seeks to assess. An important tenet of an RCT is that it attempts to control variables to enhance the researcher's ability to assess the impact of the intervention. This is accomplished by assigning participants randomly, blinding the participants (and the assessors when practical) to the conditions, and mitigating items that would confound the results.[4]

CATs are brief documents created by clinicians to quickly share the outcomes of appraised studies with other clinicians. These are defined further in chapter 6. Systematic reviews analyze quality studies published in the literature related to a question of interest. They are intended to be all-inclusive reviews of relevant literature addressing a question of interest. A meta-analysis uses statistical methods to assess the quality of published studies or to compare the statistical results of numerous published studies. The goal is to lead to increased strength in recommendations that may relate to how ATs treat certain medical conditions. An MA may analyze a series of RCTs on a particular topic (e.g., the impact of NSAIDs on gastrointestinal irritation) to evaluate the RCTs for rigor in explaining variations in outcomes.[4] In the profession of athletic training, the National Athletic Trainers' Association (NATA) position statements incorporate SAs and MAs to inform those in the profession about best practices based on the current available evidence. These techniques are further explained in chapter 6.

The final three items you will note on the pyramid are references to unfiltered information, filtered information, and the TRIP Database. The TRIP Database is a medical search engine that requires registration; a standard membership search is free, but options are limited. TRIP uses an algorithm to search both filtered and nonfiltered literature simultaneously. *Filtered* means that the published articles have been appraised for quality and their ability to be used as references to influence clinical practice. This is a step beyond the peer review required to publish in many journals. Unfiltered studies are published studies in the primary literature that are available from search engines such as PubMed, EBSCOhost, and others discussed in chapter 2. These may or may not have undergone peer review but have not been part of systematic reviews or appraised as part of multiple research studies and how they relate to each other in the greater picture of clinical practice.

Purpose of Evidence-Based Practice in Clinical Athletic Training

Athlete health treatment outcomes are undergoing increased scrutiny—by media outlets investigating athlete health care, those who oversee the athletic directors responsible for finances and reporting student-athlete health, the Board of Certification, and the athletes themselves. Expenses, scientific rationales, and the human outcomes of clinical practice are all being questioned. Current concussion management practices are being questioned as health care providers learn more about the long-term effects of concussions, which is driving current clinical practice in a fashion we have not previously considered on a large scale. Quality health care providers should also express a desire to improve outcomes and be interested in knowing whether the treatments they are using are truly effective and what long-term sequelae may result. It is no longer appropriate to think only about the athlete's ability to play for the remainder of the current season; we must also address the lifetime outcomes of our treatments of current conditions.

This background has resulted in a great deal of enthusiasm for EBP; however, it has hit numerous roadblocks. Practitioners often have difficulty finding and interpreting RCTs and incorporating them into their practices.[5] Many ATs lack the time to search for applicable research, and some lack the background in study appraisal or are poorly versed in understanding the statistical reporting in RCTs. The subsequent chapters will help you overcome these challenges and increase your comfort with research and your ability to find, appraise, and incorporate evidence-based research into your clinical practice. Additionally, as the profession of athletic training continues to address a desire to receive third-party reimbursement, EBP will become more important.

Summary

This chapter presented the steps required to incorporate evidence-based practice (EBP) into your treatment. It also explained the purpose behind EBP and why it is important. Health care providers are under immense scrutiny to improve outcomes and to defend the treatments they provide as beneficial and prudent. It is no longer acceptable to treat an athlete based solely on the assumption that the methods employed years ago are still adequate as our knowledge expands. As you go through the text and start to integrate evidence-based decisions into your practice, remember the important steps used to determine the impact of the evidence you read in the literature. Then never forget that the most important part of the EBP equation is the athlete. Our goal as health care providers is to provide high-quality care, keep up with the research, and listen to athletes' concerns and goals and educate them through the process of recovery.

References

1. Gray JAM, Haynes RB, Richardson WS, Rosenberg WMC, Sackett DL. Evidence based medicine: What it is and what it isn't. *Brit Med J*. 1996; 312 (7023): 71+.

2. Fetters LK, Tilson, J. *Evidence based physical therapy*. Philadelphia: Davis; 2012.

3. PEDro scale. PEDro website. www.pedro.org.au/english/downloads/pedro-scale. Accessed January 14, 2014.

4. Rosner AL. Evidence-based medicine: Revisiting the pyramid of priorities. *J Bodywork Movement Ther*. 2012; 16 (1): 42-49.

5. Brown B, Crawford P, Hicks C. *Evidence-based research: Dilemmas and debates in health care*. Glasgow: Bell and Bain; 2003.

CHAPTER 2

Steps in Evidence-Based Practice Research

Objectives

After reading this chapter, you will be able to do the following:

- Address a clinical question using a five-step process.
- Perform an evidence-based search and determine the clinical outcomes with an athlete.
- Become familiar with commonly used databases and search engines in the field of athletic training.
- Identify the common pitfalls with EBP searches and describe how to address them when they arise.

Now that you have acquired a general understanding of EBP from chapter 1, it's time to dig deeper. This chapter takes you through the steps of performing a full EBP search from start to finish. You will be guided through a five-step process and perform each step with a clinical question that interests you. At the end of the chapter, we offer some troubleshooting tips to fine-tune your future searches. The five steps in the process are as follows:

1. Create a clinically relevant and searchable question concerning your athlete.
2. Conduct a database search to find the best evidence.
3. Critically appraise the articles or evidence for quality.
4. Critically synthesize the evidence to choose and implement a treatment.
5. Assess the outcomes by monitoring the athlete.

Step 1: Create a Clinically Relevant and Searchable Question Concerning Your Athlete

Creating a clinically relevant question is often more complex than it seems. A searchable question has three or four components: the athlete or problem (or both), the intervention (treatment), often the comparison intervention (the treatment you are curious about), and the outcome measure by which the intervention is appraised. Some searches have only one intervention or comparison component.

Foundations of Evidence: Components of a Searchable Question

1. Athlete or problem (or both)
2. Intervention or treatment
3. Comparison intervention
4. Outcome

To begin the process, consider your current clinical work with athletes. If a particular case you are working with is complex or difficult, consider using that for your question. If you are not working clinically, consider an injury, illness, or treatment you would like to learn more about. If you are having a hard time coming up with something, here are a few scenarios to consider:

• **Scenario A:** A young female soccer player is returning to play after a six-month rehab program following an ACL tear. She had a bone-patellar tendon-bone (BPTB) graft to reconstruct the ACL, which is creating some minor residual anterior pain. In the first game back, she suffers an ACL tear in the opposite knee. Given the residual pain from the first ACL surgery, she asks you whether an allograft is a better option for the second knee reconstruction. You decide to do an EBP search to address her question.

• **Scenario B:** A young male basketball player has been battling chronic Achilles tendinosis for 10 months and is getting frustrated. A colleague shared a similar case with you and suggested adding eccentric exercises to the rehab plan. You decide to do an EBP search to determine whether there is any increased risk of rupture when adding eccentrics to a chronic Achilles tendon injury.

• **Scenario C:** You walk out to track practice one day and are alarmed that a quarter of your athletes have applied kinesiology tape in various places on their legs. Some of your colleagues have reported gains from the use of kinesiology tape, whereas others claim that it is a money-making scheme and doesn't work beyond the placebo effect. You decide to do an EBP search to find out whether kinesiology tape is proven to reduce injury symptoms.

To structure your EBP question, you need to put it into the **PICO** format:

P: *Patient* (or athlete) and *problem* (or injury)

I: *Intervention* currently in place

C: *Comparison* intervention

O: *Outcome* to measure to determine which intervention is best for the athlete

Defining P is the easy step. This is your athlete (and perhaps the sport, the position, or both) and the athlete's injury, illness, or condition. Avoid being too detailed initially. For example, you may want to avoid limiting age beyond, say, *youth* or *geriatric*. However, you should state the exact injury or condition (e.g., *patellar tendinitis* rather than *knee injury*). The latter would garner thousands of articles. For scenario A, the P would be female soccer athletes with ACL tears. You would not want to enter *collegiate*, because doing so may limit the results, and this categorization is less important. However, *female* is an important word to include, given the disparities between male and female ACL injury rates. Now consider the scenario from your clinical practice, and write your patient and problem on a separate piece of paper.

Now it's time to define I. The intervention is most commonly what is already present—a current treatment, the surgery that has been chosen, or anything along those lines. If I is a regular rehabilitation protocol, you may compare it with the C treatment that uses the same regular rehabilitation protocol plus iontophoresis, for example. The I would be the treatment you are currently providing or the surgery commonly performed. In the research studies you find in your search, this I group may be the control group, meaning the group that underwent the normal treatment or surgery. For scenario A, the intervention would be autograft ACL surgery. You may want to define the type of graft, such as bone-patellar tendon-bone (BPTB) or hamstring. In many scenarios, the intervention may be a normal treatment—nothing new. For example, for acute patellar tendinitis, the I may be providing a normal treatment and *not* stretching the quadriceps, whereas the C may be providing a normal treatment and adding an aggressive quad stretching component. For scenario C, the intervention would be providing a normal treatment and *not* applying kinesiology tape. Now consider the scenario from your clinical practice, and write your intervention on a separate piece of paper.

To define C, consider the new comparison intervention that you are wondering about. This is most commonly the real point of your EBP question—that is, is there something better out there than what you are doing or intend to do? In most of the research articles you will find in your search, this group will be the experimental group, meaning the group that received the extra treatment, new surgery, or the like. For scenario A, the comparison would be allograft ACL surgery. For scenario C, the C would be applying the kinesiology tape while doing the normal rehab on any injuries. Now consider the scenario from your clinical practice, and write your comparison on a separate piece of paper.

The last step in creating a searchable question is defining the outcome measure (O), or what you intend to look at to see which I or C is best for your athlete. Many times in athletic training, the outcome may be time to return to play or reinjury rate. Other common outcome measures are pain level, reduction of symptoms, and range of motion. At times, you may need to get into the research studies to find out what is most commonly used as the outcome measure for the issue you are investigating. For example, if you are wondering whether acromioclavicular surgery is as effective as conservative, nonsurgical rehabilitation treatment, your outcome variable could be how quickly people return to play or how often people in each group become reinjured. The determination of which outcome measure to use in your search may be dictated by your athlete's values or priorities or by whatever you find in your search. Is your athlete more concerned with getting back to play quickly or getting back to play safely with little chance of reinjury? For scenario A (ACL graft options), the outcome measure needs to take into consideration what the athlete is concerned about—specifically, the amount of residual pain she had after her first BPTB autograft surgery. For that search, the outcome would be pain level postsurgery. For scenario C (kinesiology tape), the outcome would be reduction of symptoms. Now consider the scenario from your clinical practice, and write your outcome on a separate piece of paper.

Now it's time to put your full PICO question together from the components that you wrote on the piece of paper. Be sure to read variations of the question out loud to hear what arrangement of the PICO sounds most appropriate. For scenario A with the ACL, the question may be stated like this: For female soccer players with ACL tears, does a BPTB autograft or an allograft create less postsurgical pain through RTP (return to play)? For scenario B with the Achilles tendon, the question may be stated in this way: For male basketball players with chronic Achilles tendon injuries, is the risk of rupture increased when adding eccentrics to the rehabilitation program? And for scenario C with the kinesiology tape, the question may be stated in this way: For running athletes with orthopedic injuries, does the application of kinesiology tape create a more rapid reduction of symptoms than not using the tape?

Now that you have created your PICO question, you are ready to hit the computer to start your search. If you are missing components of PICO, you may have created a nonsearchable EBP question. Also, a question that asks simple demographic or statistical questions may be nonsearchable. For example, whether rugby players or American football players get more concussions is simply an epidemiological statistic and not a question that involves interventions. Finally, if your outcome measure is not quantifiable, you need to revise it to make it more refined. For example, if your PICO is comparing two surgeries to see which is "better" as the outcome measure, you will likely find no articles, because no research articles use the undefined term *better* as the outcome. See the sidebar Examples of Searchable and Nonsearchable EBP Questions.

Step 2: Conduct a Database Search to Find the Best Evidence

This step is new to many clinicians. Although most of us may keep up on reading one or two journals that pertain to our profession, literally hundreds of health care–related journals may contain evidence to help us answer our questions. Learning how to navigate and tap into those resources can be daunting.

Search Engines and Databases

Numerous search engines and databases are available to filter those thousands of journal titles for you. **Databases** are online collections of research articles, whereas **search engines** are tools used to search one or more databases. Medline is one of

Examples of Searchable and Nonsearchable EBP Questions

Searchable Questions

Patient and problem: Track sprinters with medial tibial stress syndrome (MTSS)

Intervention: Rehabilitation and rest

Comparison: Rehabilitation and kinesiology tape

Outcome: Pain reduction

Question: Do track sprinters with MTSS have greater pain reduction with rehabilitation and rest or with rehabilitation and kinesiology tape?

Patient and problem: Female soccer players

Intervention: Core stability ACL injury prevention program

Comparison: Jump landing ACL injury prevention program

Outcome: Occurrences of ACL tears

Question: In female soccer players, is there a reduced incidence of ACL tears for those performing core stability programs compared with those performing jump landing programs?

Nonsearchable Questions

Patient and problem: Athletes with MTSS

Intervention: No treatment, or rest

Comparison:

Outcome: Ability to complete the season

Question: Are athletes with MTSS able to complete the season?

Patient and problem: Soccer players

Intervention: Core strengthening programs

Comparison:

Outcome: Improved performance

Question: Do soccer players who perform core strengthening programs have improved soccer performance?

the most comprehensive databases available in health care and medicine; PubMed, one of the most powerful search engines, searches Medline and a host of other databases. Figure 2.1 shows the PubMed database page where you would begin a search by typing in your PICO components.[1] Figure 2.2 shows the Cochrane Library database initial search page.[2] **Preappraised resources** are databases that contain

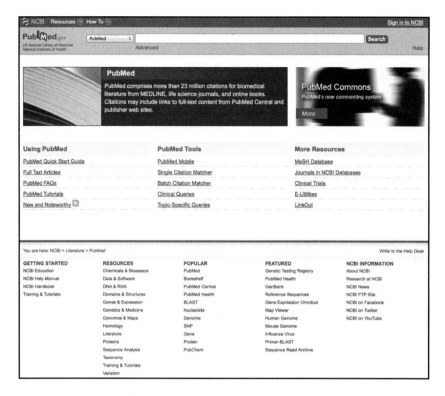

Figure 2.1 PubMed database initial search page.

Reprinted from PubMed.gov. Available: www.ncbi.nlm.nih.gov/pubmed.

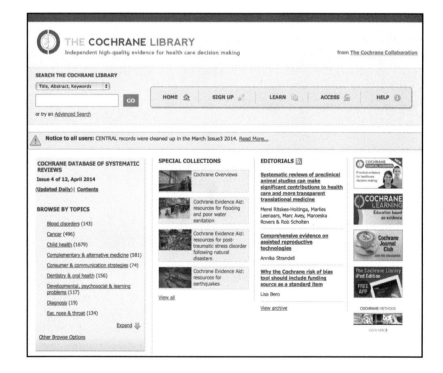

Figure 2.2 Cochrane Library database initial search page.

Reprinted from The Cochrane Library. Available: www.thecochranelibrary.com/view/0/index.html.

research that has already been at least minimally evaluated for quality. These resource databases, however, contain far fewer research articles than PubMed or the Cochrane Library. **Metasearch engines** present only meta-analyses, which are discussed in chapter 6. TRIP (Translating Research Into Practice) is one of the most powerful search engines for medical practitioners; it searches numerous databases to find the best available **evidence** for clinical practice.

Search engines and databases are usually available at university and college library research links from library web pages. See the sidebar Relevant Health Care Databases and Search Engines. Go to each of these websites and get an idea of what they are about and how they are organized. Some require you to set up a user account at no cost. This allows you to save search keywords and articles, per search.

Relevant Health Care Databases and Search Engines

Databases and Search Engines

PubMed

Cochrane Library

Centre for Reviews and Dissemination (CRD)

Database of Abstracts of Reviews of Effects (DARE)

Cumulative Index to Nursing and Allied Health (CINAHL)

Meta-Search Engine

TRIP

Preappraised Resources

ACP Journal Club

Clinical Evidence

DynaMed

Essential Evidence Plus

FPIN Clinical Inquiries

UpToDate

Application of PICO Searching

To get started with your EBP search from the PICO question you created, go to the PubMed search engine. At the initial search page, enter your PICO components as keywords in the search box at the top of the web page (see figure 2.3 for an illustration of where to enter your PICO). Remember to use Boolean operators (discussed later in this chapter) as appropriate. As an example, the keywords for a search may look like the following, from which you can gain an understanding of the full PICO question: *soccer players AND ACL surgery AND autograft OR allograft AND pain*. Now

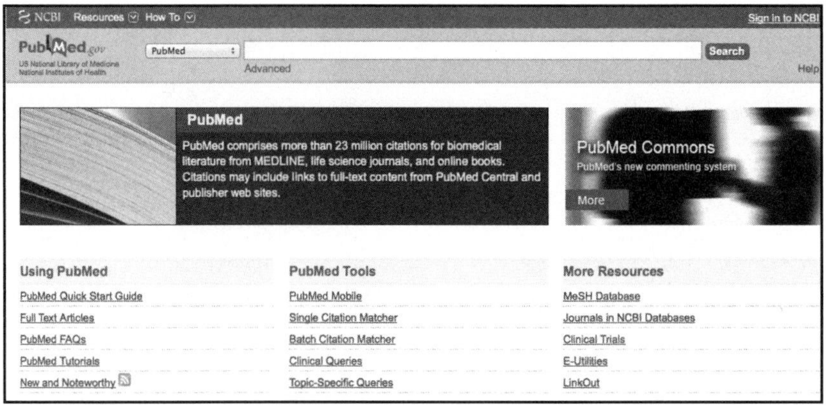

Figure 2.3 Close-up of PubMed search page keyword input area.
Reprinted from PubMed.gov. Available: www.ncbi.nlm.nih.gov/pubmed.

hit the search button. If your search returns zero hits, you have likely entered search terms that are too narrow. Consider broadening your terms, perhaps using the OR Boolean operator word. If your search returns over a couple of hundred articles, you have likely not narrowed down your search terms enough. Consider being more specific with your P, I, C, or O—use specific words rather than concept terms. For example, rather than entering *rehabilitation,* you may want to enter *strength exercises.* Once you believe that you have a good group of articles that directly address your question, it is time to enter step 3 of the search process. You should have two to six articles that directly address your PICO question.

Search Techniques

You need to know how to best type in your question once you find the database you want to search (which is covered in the next section). This is called the search technique. Each database presents various views with boxes in which to enter the keywords of your PICO question. The danger of not using a search technique is that you may end up with thousands of articles. Using a search technique allows you to narrow the scope of the search up front to avoid having to sift through those thousands of articles one by one. You will get better at this with practice. The two most common search techniques are the Boolean search and the subject or medical subject heading search.

Boolean Search

The **Boolean search** technique requires the strategic use of the words *AND, OR,* and *NOT* when inputting your question. These three operator words will help specify a complex EBP question to provide usable results. The *OR* operator is used when you need a broader search that includes either of two words, typically. For example, you could use *autograft OR allograft* to search for articles on either ACL surgical technique. This would result in hundreds of results. To narrow that down, you may want to use the *AND* operator. This command creates a search that pulls up only articles that have both of the words in the title. For example, you could use *autograft AND allograft* to find articles that address both surgical techniques

Boolean Modifiers at a Glance

Boolean modifier	When to use	Example	Function
AND	When you want results that include both search terms	autograft AND allograft	Limits search
OR	When you want results that include either search term	autograft OR allograft	Expands search
NOT	When you want results that include the first search term but not the second	anterior cruciate NOT posterior cruciate	Limits search
Phrase	When you want to find your search term as an exact phrase	"hamstring autograft"	Limits search

in the same paper. The third operator in a Boolean search, *NOT,* can narrow your search even further, if warranted. Use *NOT* to exclude articles that have that word in the title or abstract. Be careful here. If you use *NOT* for a general word, such as *posterior* to rule out posterior cruciate hits from your anterior cruciate search, you will rule out any article that refers to anything posterior. So be specific, such as *anterior cruciate NOT posterior cruciate.* This way, only articles about the posterior cruciate ligament will be excluded. Although we use the operators *OR* and *AND* often, *NOT* is used much less frequently in searches.

Subject or Medical Subject Heading Search

The medical subject heading search is called a **MeSH search**.[1] This technique is used when you are in certain medical databases and require a broader search. The databases have a list of medical headings to choose from. You can scroll down and click on any number of medical topics to start your search (figure 2.4). For example, if you want to search a specific treatment for patellar tendinitis, you would use the MeSH headings *tendinopathy* and *knee.* The problem with MeSH headings is that you cannot be very specific, which is often needed with EBP searches. So, do not be alarmed if your first attempt at using MeSH headings yields results that are not specific to your question. Using MeSH headings takes practice.

Step 3: Critically Appraise the Articles or Evidence for Quality

Once you have a sufficient number of directly related articles, it's time to start reading those that are most closely related to your question. The results page will list the title, authors, and all other citation information (figure 2.5). From the titles, you can click on the most relevant to read the full abstract (figure 2.6). From the abstract, you can click again to either see the full text or find out where you can retrieve it. Often, reading the abstract will give you enough information to determine whether the full text will help you with your clinical question.

Unfortunately, many research articles are published without thorough reviews to determine the quality of the research. Thus, it is incumbent upon you to determine

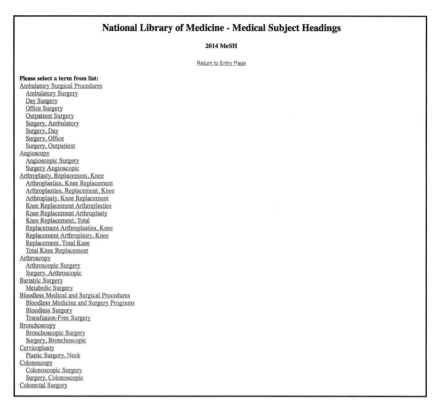

Figure 2.4 MeSH headings initial search page showing heading options.
Reprinted from PubMed.gov. Available: www.ncbi.nlm.nih.gov/pubmed.

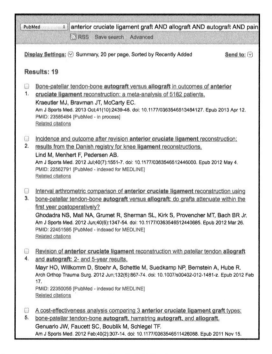

Figure 2.5 Initial search results page in PubMed.
Reprinted from PubMed.gov. Available: www.ncbi.nlm.nih.gov/pubmed.

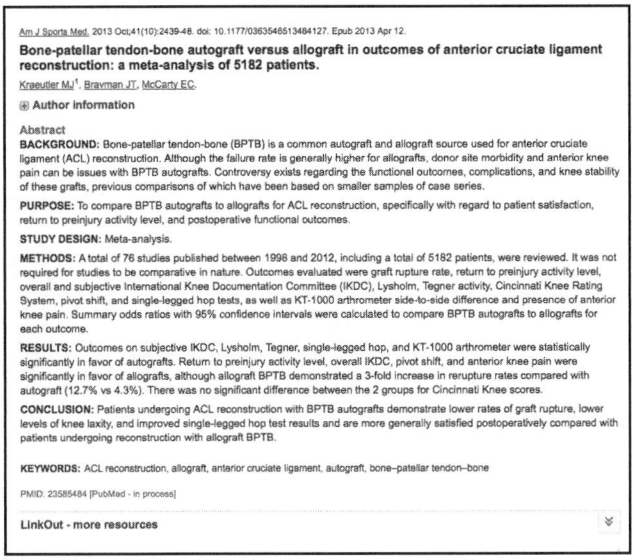

Am J Sports Med. 2013 Oct;41(10):2439-48. doi: 10.1177/0363546513484127. Epub 2013 Apr 12.

Bone-patellar tendon-bone autograft versus allograft in outcomes of anterior cruciate ligament reconstruction: a meta-analysis of 5182 patients.

Kraeutler MJ[1], Bravman JT, McCarty EC.

⊕ Author information

Abstract

BACKGROUND: Bone-patellar tendon-bone (BPTB) is a common autograft and allograft source used for anterior cruciate ligament (ACL) reconstruction. Although the failure rate is generally higher for allografts, donor site morbidity and anterior knee pain can be issues with BPTB autografts. Controversy exists regarding the functional outcomes, complications, and knee stability of these grafts, previous comparisons of which have been based on smaller samples of case series.

PURPOSE: To compare BPTB autografts to allografts for ACL reconstruction, specifically with regard to patient satisfaction, return to preinjury activity level, and postoperative functional outcomes.

STUDY DESIGN: Meta-analysis.

METHODS: A total of 76 studies published between 1998 and 2012, including a total of 5182 patients, were reviewed. It was not required for studies to be comparative in nature. Outcomes evaluated were graft rupture rate, return to preinjury activity level, overall and subjective International Knee Documentation Committee (IKDC), Lysholm, Tegner activity, Cincinnati Knee Rating System, pivot shift, and single-legged hop tests, as well as KT-1000 arthrometer side-to-side difference and presence of anterior knee pain. Summary odds ratios with 95% confidence intervals were calculated to compare BPTB autografts to allografts for each outcome.

RESULTS: Outcomes on subjective IKDC, Lysholm, Tegner, single-legged hop, and KT-1000 arthrometer were statistically significantly in favor of autografts. Return to preinjury activity level, overall IKDC, pivot shift, and anterior knee pain were significantly in favor of allografts, although allograft BPTB demonstrated a 3-fold increase in rerupture rates compared with autograft (12.7% vs 4.3%). There was no significant difference between the 2 groups for Cincinnati Knee scores.

CONCLUSION: Patients undergoing ACL reconstruction with BPTB autografts demonstrate lower rates of graft rupture, lower levels of knee laxity, and improved single-legged hop test results and are more generally satisfied postoperatively compared with patients undergoing reconstruction with allograft BPTB.

KEYWORDS: ACL reconstruction, allograft, anterior cruciate ligament, autograft, bone–patellar tendon–bone

PMID: 23585484 [PubMed - in process]

LinkOut - more resources ⌄

Figure 2.6 Detailed abstract from a results page article.
Reprinted from PubMed.gov. Available: www.ncbi.nlm.nih.gov/pubmed.

whether the research articles you find in step 2 are well done in terms of methods and conclusions. Evaluating (appraising) research articles can be difficult. Thus, we have devoted chapters 4 and 5 to creating critical appraisal outlines to assist you. Scales have also been developed to help clinicians evaluate research articles. Here are two examples:

- Oxford Centre for Evidence-Based Medicine scale[4] (figure 2.7)
- Physiotherapy Evidence Database scale (PEDro)[3] (figure 2.8)

These scales offer standard criteria for critical appraisal.

With these resources and what you will learn in chapters 4 and 5, you will be able to adequately evaluate research articles. As you gain more practice with these appraisals, it will become easier to determine research quality when reading the articles. Additionally, learning the basics of research methods and statistical analysis, as presented in chapter 3, will assist in your appraisals. Once you have your top two to six articles that directly answer your PICO question and have met your preferred appraisal quality, it is time to determine exactly what to do with what you've discovered.

Don't be alarmed if the results of your articles do not match. For example, in our kinesiology tape example, you may have articles that report that the tape reduces injury symptoms and others that report that it does not. When this disparity occurs, the critical appraisal of each article becomes paramount. For example, the articles that report positive results may have had no control group, meaning there was only one experimental group and no other group to compare it with. Conversely, the articles that report no effect of kinesiology taping may have had an experimental group that received kinesiology tape and a control group that received a placebo tape that looked like kinesiology tape, both of which reported a

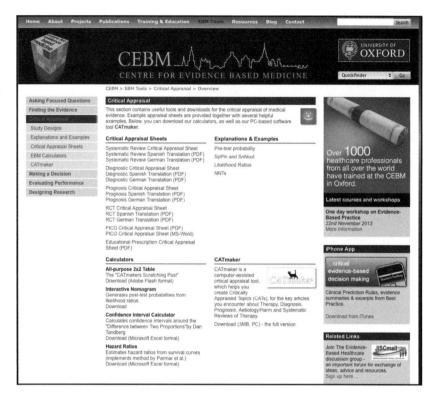

Figure 2.7 Oxford Centre for Evidence-Based Medicine scales for critical appraisal.
Reprinted from Oxford Centre for Evidence Based Medicine Scale.

decrease in injury symptoms. Thus, no significant difference was found between groups. This would be the more well-designed study and thus the one that you should consider the outcomes.

Step 4: Critically Synthesize the Evidence to Choose and Implement a Treatment

After reviewing the quality of your top two to six articles, it's time to apply your findings with your athlete. It is good practice to share your EBP search results with your athletes, because it lets them know that you care about them and want to give them the best possible care. If your results are mixed—even with great research quality in all of your final articles—then that is exactly what you report to your athlete. Explain that more research needs to be done in that area. If, after all of your search efforts, you find that your question has not been researched (meaning there is no evidence on the topic), then that is fine to share with your athlete also. More often than not, though, you will find a clear answer to your PICO question.

When it comes time to choose a treatment, you must consider the needs of your athlete. Recall that EBP is a combination of evidence, athlete needs, and clinician

PEDro Scale

1. Eligibility criteria were specified.   No ☐   Yes ☐
   Where: _____

2. Subjects were randomly allocated to groups (in a crossover study, subjects were randomly allocated an order in which treatments were received).   No ☐   Yes ☐
   Where: _____

3. Allocation was concealed.   No ☐   Yes ☐
   Where: _____

4. The groups were similar at baseline regarding the most important prognostic indicators.   No ☐   Yes ☐
   Where: _____

5. There was blinding of all subjects.   No ☐   Yes ☐
   Where: _____

6. There was blinding of all therapists who administered the therapy.
   No ☐   Yes ☐
   Where: _____

7. There was blinding of all assessors who measured at least one key outcome.   No ☐   Yes ☐
   Where: _____

8. Measures of at least one key outcome were obtained from more than 85% of the subjects initially allocated to groups.   No ☐   Yes ☐
   Where: _____

9. All subjects for whom outcome measures were available received the treatment or control condition as allocated or, where this was not the case, data for at least one key outcome were analyzed by "intention to treat."   No ☐   Yes ☐
   Where: _____

10. The results of between-group statistical comparisons are reported for at least one key outcome.   No ☐   Yes ☐
    Where: _____

11. The study provides both point measures and measures of variability for at least one key outcome.   No ☐   Yes ☐
    Where: _____

Figure 2.8   Physiotherapy Evidence Database scale (PEDro). Visit the PEDro website to understand how to use and read the outcomes of this scale.
Reprinted from PEDro.org.

experience. To this point, you've gathered the evidence and considered your clinical experiences. Now you must be certain that your treatment of choice falls in line with your athlete's needs or values (or both). For example, should the female soccer player with a second ACL tear have surgery immediately, or is it OK for her to wait until after the Thanksgiving holiday? Family support may be more important to her than having the surgery immediately. These considerations, which are unique to your athlete, are not in the evidence databases, but they are equally important. The best clinicians naturally keep their athletes' needs front and center when making treatment decisions. Once you and your athlete have determined the treatment of choice and implemented the plan, you begin step 5.

Step 5: Assess the Outcomes by Monitoring the Athlete

After you have weighted your EBP search outcomes, your clinical experiences, and your athlete's needs and implemented the treatment of choice, it's time to evaluate whether the treatment was effective. What are the results? Are the results reproducible and valid? Does your athlete feel positive about the treatment outcomes? Has the condition, problem, injury, or illness been ameliorated?

When we assess outcomes, we look at whether the results are disease or injury oriented or athlete oriented (or both)—that is, we measure the effectiveness of the treatment based on whether the athlete got better or feels better or positive about the treatment. It is one thing to note whether the athlete got better, but it is another to compare your outcomes with the norm, or the outcomes of other athletes. Several outcome constructs have been developed to assist in making comparisons. The following five general constructs may be considered with clinical outcomes assessment:

Disablement theory—athlete oriented

Health-related quality of life—athlete oriented

Global rating of change—both athlete and injury oriented

Minimal clinically important difference—injury oriented

Minimal detectable difference—injury oriented

- **Disablement theory** proposes that acute and chronic injury or illness affects the body's systems—physical and mental—thereby affecting activities of daily living.[5] Personal and environmental factors (risk factors, interventions, and stressors) can either speed or slow recovery. You should continually be cognizant of how being injured and progressing through rehabilitation are affecting the athlete both in and out of the athletic training room or clinic.

- **Health-related quality of life** is similar to disablement theory in that physical and mental health perceptions (health risks and conditions, functional status, social support, and socioeconomic status) are proposed to affect the outcome of injury.[6] Athletes come into our care with unique backgrounds and expectations, all of which may affect treatment outcomes. Our task is to restore their health-related quality of life to preinjury status or better.

- **Global rating of change (GRC)** measures a combination of athlete satisfaction and injury improvement from the athlete's viewpoint.[7] GRC uses athlete-rated change as an outcome measure to determine the efficacy of a rehabilitation plan, progression, or treatment. The athlete rates the treatment on a quantifiable scale.

- **Minimal clinically important difference (MCID)** and **minimal detectable difference (MDC)** are quantifiable ratings that report the effectiveness of the treatment in terms of injury improvement from the athlete's viewpoint, most commonly.[7] Minimal clinically important differences (MCID) are athlete-derived scores that reflect changes in injury status from a clinical intervention that are meaningful for the athlete. Many methods are used to obtain an MCID, which may cause difficulties in comparing studies.

Regardless of which outcome construct you follow, step 5 requires you to evaluate the treatment you implemented. Be sure to evaluate both injury improvement (hopefully) and the athlete's impression of progress. If your treatment was not as effective as you had anticipated, then you may need to get back into EBP search mode to find something more effective. If you had great outcomes, you should consider your first EBP trial a great success. Our hope is that the more you practice the five-step process, the faster you will navigate it.

Search Troubleshooting Tips

Numerous problems may occur with EBP searching. One of the most common for new EBP searchers is thinking in terms of concepts rather than specific words when inputting the initial search.[8] If you put in a grand concept term, such as *rehabilitation*, your results could number in the hundreds of thousands and include mental rehab, drug rehab, and animal rehab. Use specific words instead, such as *patellar tendon rehabilitation*, *rotator cuff rehabilitation*, or *concussion rehabilitation*.

Consider refining your search terms if you find too many or too few articles. If too few articles show up in your results, you will likely need to broaden your search terms by using fewer patient or problem words. For example, if you input the term *collegiate women's soccer players with ACL tears*, you could broaden the search by using *soccer players with ACL tears*. You may also want to use a Boolean operator in your search, such as *soccer AND anterior cruciate ligament tears*.

If too many articles show up in your results, you likely need to use more specific terms. For example, if you input *Achilles tendon rehabilitation*, you could pare down your search by being more specific with *Achilles tendon AND eccentric exercises*.

Always remember that not every aspect of injury and treatment in athletic training has been studied. So do not be surprised if there is no evidence about a clinical question that you investigate. A fruitful thing to do when you find an article that answers your question is to look through the reference list at the end of that article. Even if you find only one article that answers your clinical question and it is of good quality, the reference list may provide more directly relevant articles.

Summary

This chapter provided more in-depth knowledge about creating and investigating a searchable PICO clinical question. You were guided through a five-step process of EBP searching. You created your own PICO question and used that question to perform a full evidence search, hopefully to reveal articles that directly answered your question. Several database search engines were presented for future use, along with strategies to refine your search techniques. Performing a critical appraisal of the evidence is a difficult arena for many clinicians, which is why chapters 4 and 5 go into more depth beyond the general information on critical appraisal presented here. With quality evidence in hand, you were then guided through choosing and implementing a treatment for your athlete. Several clinical outcome assessment tools were then discussed to help you evaluate the efficacy of the newly implemented treatment. The chapter concluded with some EBP search troubleshooting tips to keep in mind for future searches.

References

1. PubMed website. www.ncbi.nlm.nih.gov/pubmed. Accessed April 4, 2014.

2. Cochrane Library website. www.thecochranelibrary.com/view/0/index.html. Accessed April 4, 2014.

3. PEDro scale. PEDro website. www.pedro.org.au/english/downloads/pedro scale. Accessed January 14, 2014.

4. Oxford Centre for Evidence-Based Medicine (CEBM) scale. Centre for Evidence-Based Medicine website. www.cebm.net/index.aspx?o=1157. Accessed January 14, 2014.

5. Vela LI, Denegar C. Transient disablement in the physically active with musculoskeletal injuries, part I: A descriptive model. *J Athl Train*. 2010; 45 (6): 615-629.

6. Learmonth Y, Hubbard E, McAuley E, Motl R. Psychometric properties of quality of life and health-related quality of life assessments in people with multiple sclerosis. *Qual Life Res*. 2014; ePub ahead of print.

7. King M. A point of minimal important difference (MID): A critique of terminology and methods. *Outcomes Res*. 2011; 11 (2): 171-184.

8. Fetters LK, Tilson J. *Evidence based physical therapy*. Philadelphia: Davis; 2012.

CHAPTER 3

Research Evaluation

Objectives

After reading this chapter, you will be able to do the following:

- Identify and describe forms of reliability used to assess research for use in evidence-based practice.
- Differentiate between validity and reliability.
- Understand the importance of and aspects of prevalence testing.
- Apply sensitivity and specificity in your practice and selection of special tests.

Everything that involves research revolves around questions and unknowns. Research is a search for answers through trial and speculation. Nothing in research is certain; we want to make educated decisions and reach reasonable conclusions. Research outcomes often only support or fail to support a proposed treatment or assessment method; rarely, if ever, would we say the method is proven. Because the methods used to treat injuries and illnesses continue to evolve, so must the evidence-based clinician. At one time, the preferred method to clean a wound was to use hydrogen peroxide. Now we realize that hydrogen peroxide destroys healthy cells; newer cleaning methods such as saline and betadine are less caustic to healthy tissue. Ten years ago it was not uncommon to assess an athlete on the sideline after a suspected concussion and return him to play the same day, but newer evidence no longer supports same-day return. Thus, as evidence advances, so should your practice. In the meantime, as an evidence-based clinician, you need to make sure that the assessments you use are as accurate as possible.

Reliability

The first term that is important for a consumer of research to understand is reliability. By strict definition, **reliability** refers to consistency in measures attained by people or instruments.[1,2] Basically, does the tool you are using produce the same outcome each time you use it? An easy example is a pair of tape cutters. If every time you use the cutters to remove tape, you achieve a nice, clean cut, you would consider these cutters reliable. However, if sometimes they cut the tape and other times they do not, you would never know what outcome to expect; you would therefore consider these cutters unreliable. Reliability is important when you are trying to make a clinical decision. If you are performing an anterior drawer test on an ankle and one time you perform the test you feel laxity and the next time you fail to feel laxity, you will have difficulty making a decision. You may question whether the athlete changed, whether you applied different degrees of force, or whether the test itself is unreliable.

Reliability also relates to questionnaires. A well-structured item on a questionnaire should be easy to understand and not subject to misinterpretation. Let's look at an example of an item that uses a **Likert scale** of 1 to 4, with 1 being low or disagree and 4 being high or strongly agree. Here is the statement: *Some of the most important tasks of an athletic trainer are administration duties and the bidding process.* Although we can all agree that athletic trainers (ATs) often have some administrative duties and likely need to bid on purchases, this is a poor item that would probably be unreliable. One reader might believe that the most important duties of an AT relate to prevention and mark 1 for this item. Another reader might focus on the bidding portion of the statement and, believing that it's not that important, also mark 1. The researcher in this case has a value of 1 on two occasions but for very different reasons. However, an AT with administrative duties might focus on the administrative portion of the statement and rate this a 4. These varied scores based on individual interpretations of the statement would lead to low reliability and prohibit the researcher from drawing a valid conclusion.

Perhaps a better statement would look like this: *Athletic trainers should have administrative skills.* The scores for this may also vary, but they are less likely to vary because of misinterpretation. The variance in the scores would most likely be due to a variance in the opinions of the respondents. Thus, it is important to know that a study you are reviewing reports reliability values; without them, it's very difficult to trust the findings and make a judgment based on them.

You should be minimally familiar with several types of reliability measures as an evidence-based clinician. Presented here are four primary types: internal reliability, test–retest reliability, interrater reliability, and intrarater reliability.

Internal Reliability

Internal reliability is often an issue with surveys and questionnaires that employ a Likert scale system of values. The researcher wants to know whether the participant is responding to similar questions consistently. That is, did the person answer different questions about the same topic or construct in a similar manner?[1] Let's assume that the researcher has a 30-item survey to find out athletes' opinions of the school's coaching staff. On item 4, which states that the school's coaching staff sincerely cares about athletes, an athlete might respond with a 1 (low or disagree). However, item 22 asks whether the athlete agrees that the coaches exhibit a caring nature; the athlete might score this item as a 4 (high or strongly agree). This is an example of two items asking about the same construct and receiving two very different responses, when the researcher would expect these answers to be similar. However, just because one person completes a survey in this fashion does not mean that the survey is unreliable. Only if a large number of participants answer the survey in this fashion would it be considered low in internal reliability. This indicates that the sample population misunderstood the items, they deliberately answered in an odd fashion, or the items need to be dropped or reworded to increase consistency. This touches on one assumption of survey research, which is that participants answer honestly.

Test–Retest Reliability

The next form of reliability is **test–retest reliability**. As the name implies, it entails administering the test or assessment on more than one occasion. Test–retest reliability refers to the ability of an instrument or assessment to produce similar outcomes in the same group of people on multiple occasions in an amount of time that would not lead to a change in the measurement of interest.[1,2] Let's assume that you use a dynamometer to assess the triceps extension strength in a group of athletes. The athletes are healthy college males between 18 and 24 years of age who are free of injury or disease and not participating in a strength training program. You would not expect their triceps strength to change in a week's time. It is safe to assume that the scores of the first test and those of the second test will be similar. In this case, large changes in strength measures are likely due to unreliable measures being detected by the dynamometer or test administrator error.

Not all test–retest measures are as easy to visualize or straightforward as the strength testing example. If you take a standardized test such as the SAT or GRE twice, a week apart, and you don't study between the tests, your scores will likely be similar. That's because taking a large standardized test covering topics you might not know won't teach you the topics. If a person scores low in algebra on the SAT, merely taking the SAT again won't improve his ability to apply algebra. This is not the case with certain types of cognitive assessment. A standard practice for the assessment of concussion often includes a computerized concussion assessment. These types of tests, however, result in athletes learning how to take the test, subsequently increasing their scores on follow-up trials. This is referred to as a **practice effect**.

Two of the most common cognitive-based tests in clinical athletic training practice are the ImPACT Concussion Management Software (ImPACT Applications, Pittsburgh, PA) and Concussion Sentinel (CogState Ltd, Victoria, Australia). These tests present with low to moderate test–retest reliability. This means that the scores of participants completing the assessments varied more than what is considered acceptable between tests, which diminishes their clinical relevance. Test–retest reliability is often reported in the literature as a value between 0 and 1, with value of 1 being more reliable or having fewer random effects that are unaccounted for in the results.[3] The closer these reported values are to 1, the more reliable the assessments are, or the more trust you can put in them.

Interrater Reliability

Consensus between professionals on how to best treat an injury is important. It does, however, require that similar results or conditions be interpreted the same way. If you are an experienced AT reviewing injury reports upon returning to work after a few days off, you want to trust that other ATs completed certain orthopedic assessments the same way you would. More important, you hope that those tests

Foundations of Evidence: Test–Retest Reliability

When referencing test–retest reliability, a value of 0 means that no reliability or correlation existed between the tests. A score of 1 means that a perfect correlation existed between the tests. Reliability in this sense refers to whether the scores between two tests are correlated. A value of .10 would indicate a small relationship, a value of .30 would indicate a medium relationship, and values higher than .50 would indicate a large relationship and may warrant further review to determine clinical relevance.[4] The clinical relevance of values is determined based on numerous factors (e.g., time between tests, environment, maturity, effect of treatments, alternative comparisons). It is not uncommon for researchers to desire a minimum value of .60 to determine significance, which depends on numerous factors.[5]

would render the same outcome regardless of the person performing them. This is **interrater reliability**—that is, the agreement between clinicians who perform independent assessments of a condition.[6] It is important to note that the consensus should be reached by both clinicians, but independently, without cognitive influence from each other. When the second AT is assessing an injury using the same assessment as the first, she should not know the outcome of the first.[6] This ensures that the person performing the second assessment is not influenced by the outcome of the first assessment.

Also important when determining interrater reliability is that the athlete not recall the first assessment and respond differently to the second. This could be problematic when the assessment is on an injured body part and resulted in discomfort; the athlete may respond differently to the second assessment out of fear of re-creating the discomfort.

When reviewing articles and trying to determine the value of the results, remember that the higher the values for interrater reliability are, the more consistent the outcomes will be between assessors. Detailed examples are provided in subsequent chapters.

Intrarater Reliability

Intrarater reliability relates to the reproducibility of a clinical measure when performed by the same clinician on more than one occasion on the same athlete.[2] The purpose of determining intrarater reliability is to assess whether the clinician is consistently using a reliable method of assessment. If the assessment method is not established as reliable, we would return to test–retest reliability to establish trust in the assessment or instrument (recall the tape cutters). An example would be assessing the range of motion of a knee. The bony landmarks used to measure knee flexion and the mechanics of the goniometer will not change from day 1 to day 2. However, range of motion assessments often vary when repeated by the same clinician. Imagine the difficulty in creating a treatment plan when on day 1 an athlete is assessed with 100° of flexion and on day 2 has only 90° of flexion. Variations in observed outcomes will confound the care provided to athletes.

Validity

Reliability is about establishing consistent outcomes based on measures and assessments or observations. Consistent outcomes are important, as discussed in the previous section. However, what if something is consistent but not meaningful or related to real life? What if an assessment was consistent on test–retest, when different people used it, and when used over time by the same person, but it provided incorrect information? Such an assessment would be classified as invalid and therefore lacking clinical relevance. Therefore, although reliability and validity are related, they are independent.

Reliability is a precondition for validity, but its presence does not ensure validity.[1] **Validity** is best defined as the extent to which an assessment or observation measures what it is intended to measure and the extent to which that measurement is relevant.[1,2] Let's look at a simple graphic to differentiate between reliability and validity. In figure 3.1, you see three targets at which a pitcher has been throwing a ball. You are trying to establish whether he has regained control of his throwing pattern after surgery. Target *a* shows no consistent pattern or functional control of the throwing pattern and displays a lack of reliability or real-world meaning (validity). Target *b* clearly demonstrates reliable control of his throwing mechanics, but he's missing the target, or in the real world, the strike zone. This demonstrates reliability but not validity. Target *c* demonstrates that the pitcher has regained both his ability to consistently control where the ball goes and his ability to place it in a meaningful area. This demonstrates that reliability is important, but so is validity.

There are several types of validity measures, some more robust than others. Face validity, content validity, and criterion validity are discussed in the following sections.

Face Validity

The weakest type of validity is **face validity**. To report face validity, the researcher need only establish that the instrument seems to measure what it is intended to

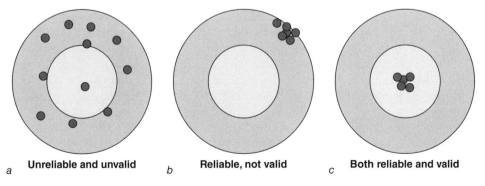

a **Unreliable and unvalid** b **Reliable, not valid** c **Both reliable and valid**

Figure 3.1 Reliability and validity pitching target.

measure.[1] Let's assume that you created an instrument to assess the pain an athlete is experiencing. This new instrument has questions on it pertaining to pain, such as When does it hurt? and Is it sharp, dull, or aching? The instrument is considered to have face validity if the researcher simply reads the questions and agrees that they relate to the construct of pain. This determination is nothing more than the opinion of the author and lacks measures of reliability. If the only validity reported for an instrument is face validity provided by the author, be reserved in your application of the instrument. A good research article will identify face validity in a statement such as this: *The researcher established face validity by having a fellow researcher review the instrument for clarity.*

Content Validity

Content validity is a slightly stronger type of validity than face validity. **Content validity** is determined when a group of experts reviews the instrument, often a questionnaire or survey, and arrives at a consensus that the instrument covers aspects of the concept it is intended to measure.[1] Returning to the example of a new pain questionnaire, the reviewers might want to see that the questions touch on numerous aspects of the pain phenomena. These might include acute pain descriptors, chronic pain descriptors, the severity of the pain, the athlete's level of anxiety, and any number of psychological variables. This could obviously be more reliable than the opinion of one author, but it still lacks pragmatic evidence. For hard, or factual, evidence to exist, there needs to be statistical analysis on the instrument or assessment; otherwise, validity is lacking.

Criterion Validity

In the realm of physical assessments, **criterion validity** is the ability of an instrument or assessment to correlate with an established assessment.[1] Evidence for criterion validity is gathered by comparing a novel assessment and an accepted method or **gold standard**. A gold standard represents measurements or assessments that are virtually undeniable.[2]

An example of a gold standard assessment is X-rays for bone fractures. When looking at the value of typical orthopedic special tests to diagnose a fracture, a tap test, squeeze test, distraction, and pressure and rotation–type test would be compared to X-rays. The more positive the correlation values are between the outcomes, the greater the criterion validity is. Values of 0 would have no correlation, and values of 1 would be perfectly correlated. Research rarely reveals a value of 0 or 1.

A description of criterion validity in the literature might appear like this: *In 847 athletes undergoing orthoscopic surgery to assess the integrity of a knee meniscus, the Thessaly test demonstrated a strong relationship (r = .87) when compared to orthopedic surgery and viewing of the meniscus.* The take-home message here is that the Thessaly test correctly indicated a torn meniscus lesion 87% of the time when compared to the gold standard.

Another example is a SLAP lesion; numerous orthopedic tests can indicate a SLAP lesion. However, the gold standard to correlate these with is arthroscopic surgery and actually being able to view the structure in question. In the absence of a gold standard assessment for comparison, a **referenced standard** can be used. A referenced standard is less indisputable than a gold standard but reasonably sufficient if justifiable.[2] An example of a referenced assessment is an MRI in the case of a SLAP lesion. It can tell the clinician more than an orthopedic test can, but it is less reliable than viewing the structure during arthroscopic surgery.

Two additional subsets of criterion validity are known-groups validity and predictive validity.[1] Both are important when making clinical decisions based on methods of assessment. **Known-groups validity** refers to the ability of an assessment to differentiate correctly between a group of people with a condition and a group of people without it.[1] Let's hypothetically consider a group of 50 people, 25 of whom have cancer and 25 of whom do not. This has been confirmed by currently acceptable methods of blood testing and CAT scan imagery. A researcher desires to test a new method to assess the presence of cancer in athletes by looking for an enzyme in saliva. The question becomes Can the new test correctly group the people with and without cancer? Its ability to correctly do this is considered its known-groups validity value.

Of course, you won't have a preexisting report on the injuries that may or may not be present in a athlete. As an evidence-based clinician, you should use tests that have been validated by researchers. The Thessaly test is a more recent method to assess a torn meniscus in the knee. It should produce different results for athletes with and without a meniscal tear. Those with a tear should have pain during the test, and those without a tear should not. If that is the case based on comparisons to an arthroscopic view of the knee, the Thessaly test would present with known-groups validity.

To have **predictive validity**, the assessment must correlate with a future event.[1] If a current assessment has a high correlation with a future event, it is predictive and potentially meaningful. To use the example of hamstring strength, quad strength of less than 50% could be correlated with future hamstring strains in athletes. If you are aware of this and your assessment has predictive validity, you can design an intervention to prevent injury. Another example is concussion management; research has shown that athletes sustaining a concussion are at greater risk for secondary injuries if they return to play too soon. The predictive validity of these studies supports conservative return-to-play guidelines.

Prevalence Independent Test

Prevalence is typically thought of as a percentage of, or the number of, people in a population who have a condition (e.g., 5 out of 100 people, or 5%). The U.S. Centers for Disease Control and Prevention (CDC) often reports the prevalence of disease in Americans. These percentages are often estimates based on a sample population. If you read a report that 7% of American adults in 2013 sustained concussions, it is highly unlikely that the CDC reviewed the medical records of every American or questioned every American. What the CDC did was sample a smaller number of people who are suspected of representing the entire population. In certain circumstances, an entire population could be sampled for a condition, resulting in a true percentage of people with the disease. For instance, a university may want to establish the prevalence of meniscal tears in all university athletes. This would require that all athletes be assessed using various methods to determine the presence of the condition. The result would be the prevalence, or the percentage, of athletes with a torn meniscus.

After properly establishing the prevalence of an injury or illness, clinicians or researchers must understand the sensitivity and specificity of the assessments they are using. Sensitivity represents the probability of a positive assessment when a condition of interest is present. Specificity represents the probability of a negative assessment when the condition of interest is absent.[7]

Accuracy

The term *accuracy* refers to a precise measure; it says that the value is true. An example is measuring the effects of ultrasound (US) on tissue temperature. If applying US at 1 MHz and 1.5 W/cm^2, we would expect a 0.3 °C/min increase in tissue temperature.[8] If you are using a thermometer to assess the increase in temperature but it records only in whole numbers, the instrument might be sensitive to an increase in temperature, but the temperature recorded may lack precision. After 2 minutes of therapy, the expected tissue temperature increase would be 0.6 °C, and the thermometer will not yet have shown an increase. After 7 minutes of treatment, the expected tissue temperature increase would be 2.1 °C, and the thermometer will show only a 2 °C increase. This example demonstrates why sensitivity and accuracy are important for clinical assessments.

Sensitivity

When determining the usefulness of an assessment, we really want to know whether it is sensitive enough to detect the injury. Will a positive sign really indicate the presence of the injury we are looking for? **Sensitivity** is the expression of how accurately an assessment can identify a problem or illness. It is determined by comparing the number of athletes who have the injury being assessed and the number of athletes who have positive findings.[6] Sensitivity is often reported as a decimal or a percentage (e.g., 85% or .85). A test reported to have a sensitivity of .78 has correctly identified a pathology 78% of the time, or correlated with the gold standard or criterion-referenced test with 78% agreement. Higher values are obviously indicative of greater sensitivity.

Sensitivity is normally established by comparing a clinical assessment with a gold standard assessment.[2] It is important to remember that there is not one cut point for a single orthopedic assessment based on just its sensitivity. Sensitivity is one part of EBP and must be weighed against the clinician's expert opinion, confidence performing an assessment, full clinical exam, and additional methods of assessment.

Let's look again at the Thessaly test for knee meniscus tears. The higher the percentage of tears the Thessaly test diagnoses compared with actually viewing the meniscus arthroscopically, the higher its sensitivity is. Various studies have reported that the Thessaly test has sensitivity values from .65 to .92, whereas the McMurray test has values from .48 to .87.[9] It could be concluded that the Thessaly test correctly diagnoses meniscus injury to a greater degree than the McMurray test does. This does not mean that as an evidence-based clinician, you won't use the McMurray test. The Thessaly test requires an athlete to stand, squat, and rotate. When this is not possible, you will need another method to assess the knee structures.[9]

Sensitivity will not always pertain to a yes-or-no diagnosis of a condition. It may also relate to change over time and whether an assessment or tool can detect that change. Let's assume that an assessment exists to depict the presence of arthritis or degenerative joint conditions. Arthritis and degenerative joint conditions would, on the surface, appear to be easily assessed. However, they are progressive and develop over time, unlike a torn ACL, which happens with the sudden anterior translation of the tibia. This prompts these questions: At what time would there be some degeneration that is not detected, and how much degeneration needs to be present for the test to assess it? Another example is the level of depression an injured athlete might experience. Many psychological assessments of depression quantify whether a person is exhibiting signs of depression. Is this same instrument capable of depicting subtle differences as the athlete remains inactive for a longer period, or if she is recovering faster than expected? Simply because an instrument has been shown to depict results on two ends of a continuum of symptoms does not ensure that it can depict subtle differences between the two extremes. In these cases, you should proceed carefully when basing your clinical decisions on sensitivity alone.

Specificity

When discussing validity, the terms *sensitivity* and *specificity* are often used together and can seem entangled. They are, however, distinctly different terms with different meanings. Sensitivity is the ability of a test to detect the true existence of an injury or condition. **Specificity** is the ability of a test or assessment to rule out an injury or condition, or to identify correctly the absence of the condition.[2] In evidence-based practice, it is important to rule out a condition to avoid treating an illness that is not present. This saves resources and time. Consider the earlier hypothetical saliva test for depicting the presence of cancer. If the test fails to correctly rule out the presence of cancer, meaning that the athlete doesn't have cancer but the test did not depict that, this athlete will undergo chemotherapy for no reason. It is important to remember that sensitivity and specificity are mutually exclusive. A test can be high in one area and low in the other. Preferred tests or assessments have moderate to high values for both sensitivity and specificity. Skilled clinicians search for two or three test that will help them rule out conditions and rule in conditions based on sensitivity and specificity scores.

Putting all this together, remember that a diagnostic test (gold standard and expensive, such as an X-ray, MRI, or arthroscopy) determines the presences or absence of a disease. ATs in field settings use less expensive screenings that might lack diagnostic values to identify injury or illness.[10] More sensitive and specific tests will enable ATs to improve their clinical diagnoses, treatments, and referrals.

Calculating Sensitivity and Specificity

To demonstrate the relationship between sensitivity and specificity, we will use a 2 × 2 table to calculate the sensitivity and specificity of a new test or one with limited diagnostic evidence compared to a gold standard. Figure 3.2 shows a positive sign (+) and a negative sign (–) under the heading of Disease, above the two columns. The positive sign (+) represents the presence of an injury or condition in real life or as depicted by a gold standard assessment. Likewise, the negative sign

(–) represents the absence of an injury or condition in real life or as depicted by a gold standard assessment. The + and – symbols at the start of the two rows and to the right of the heading New Test depict the positive test results using the new, or nondiagnostic, test for the condition or the negative results, respectively. In box A is the term **True positive**, which refers to when the new test correctly identifies a true condition depicted or confirmed by a gold standard. In box D is the term **True negative**, which occurs when the new test correctly rules out a condition that is also ruled out by a gold standard test.

Remember that if a new test indicates the presence of an injury or illness when in reality it does not exist, this would be a **false positive** finding and would be noted in box B (remember the example about being treated for cancer when the athlete does not have cancer). This is a medical error that, as an evidence-based clinician, you need to avoid. An additional error to avoid is a **false negative** (box C), which is when a new test depicts a person as not having an injury or illness when in reality the person has it. In the cancer example, a false negative test result would indicate that the athlete is free of cancer when she does in fact have cancer. As a result, the clinician fails to treat it.

The next step is to apply values to the boxes in the 2 × 2 table. Figure 3.3 is an expanded version of the 2 × 2 table. Let's assume that we are looking at ACL tears in a population of 1,000 athletes. Each athlete has been imaged with an MRI, and we know that 100 of them have ACL tears (the bottom of the + Disease column). We also know that 900 of the athletes show intact ACLs (bottom of the – Disease column). The number in box A is the number of athletes whom the new test correctly depicted as having a torn ACL (80). Box B shows the number of athletes (100) whom the new test depicted as having a torn ACL when in fact they did not. In box C we see the number of athletes (20) who have a torn ACL, but the new test failed to depict that. Finally, box D shows the number of athletes (800) whom the new test correctly depicted as not having a torn ACL.

We discussed earlier that sensitivity and specificity are different. In this 2 × 2 table, true positive conditions detected by a test (or its sensitivity) are shown in box A. The true negatives, or number of times a condition was ruled out, or the test's ability to be specific, is shown in box D, More specifically, sensitivity is box A divided

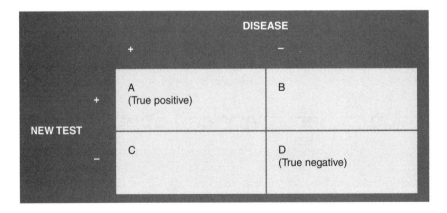

Figure 3.2   A 2 × 2 table.

		DISEASE		TOTAL
		+	−	
NEW TEST	+	A (True positive) 80	B 100	180
	−	C 20	D (True negative) 800	820
TOTAL		100	900	1000

Figure 3.3   New test (Lachman's) 2 × 2 table.

by the total of 100, or 80 / 100 = 80%. Specificity would be box D divided by 900, or 800 / 900 = 89%. Although both values are important to know and understand, how can you use these to determine the presence of a condition or if you want to trust the new test?

In our example the new test appears to have high sensitivity and specificity. At this point, you should calculate the **positive predictive value** (PPV) and **negative predictive value** (NPV) to help you assess the new test. To calculate PPV, divide box A (80) by the number of athletes the new test depicted as positive (180). The PPV is 80 / 180 = 44%; this is the percentage of times the new test correctly depicted the torn ACL. The NPV is calculated by dividing box D (800) by the number of athletes the new test depicted as not having a torn ACL (820). The NPV is 800 / 820 = 98%, which is the percentage of times the new test correctly ruled out the absence of a torn ACL.

In athletic training, assessments performed in a field setting or in an athletic training room are often not as predictive of outcomes as a gold standard test. Thus, ATs commonly perform more than one orthopedic assessment to reach a clinical decision. These are referred to as sequential assessments, and the process increases specificity.[10]

Let's use the same numbers for our first new test in figure 3.3 and add a second special test. For the sake of the example, let's classify our first test example as values determined for a Lachman's test. Based on the published PPV and NPV (the values we previously calculated) of the Lachman's test, we are not sure we can determine that our athlete truly has a torn ACL without sending him to a doctor for an MRI. At this point, it would be prudent to perform a second special test to assess the integrity of the ACL. Figure 3.4 depicts sample values for the pivot shift test on the same population of 1,000 athletes. Using the same calculations for figure 3.4 that we performed in figure 3.3, we arrive at the following values: sensitivity = 90%, specificity = 98.8%, PPV = 90%, and NPV = 98.8%.

At this point you have performed two special tests to establish the presence or absence of a torn ACL and want to know how confident you can be about this decision without sending the athlete for an MRI. This will be accomplished based on likelihood ratios and a nomogram, which are discussed next.

		DISEASE		TOTAL
		+	−	
NEW TEST	+	A (True positive) 90	B 10	100
	−	C 10	D (True negative) 890	900
TOTAL		100	900	1000

Figure 3.4 Pivot shift 2 × 2 table.

Diagnostic Accuracy

Diagnostic accuracy is a summary of measures such as the sensitivity and specificity of various tests, allowing a clinician to arrive at a conclusion. The clinician can thus inform an athlete with reasonable certainty that she does have a certain injury or illness (or reassure an athlete with reasonable certainty that she does not have a certain injury or illness). Many orthopedic apps or newer textbooks report intrarater, interrater, and test–retest values. Although they are the basis of reliability measures, they are weak measures on which to base clinical conclusions. The more appropriate measures to use when making clinical decisions are sensitivity and specificity. However, as evident in the previous section, those values alone, and the subsequent predictive values, may still leave you uncomfortable making a clinical decision without referral. You need to shift the focus of these values back to the athlete and address the issue at hand.

Likelihood Ratio

In evidence-based practice, **likelihood ratios** are easy to calculate and will help you reach conclusions pertaining to athlete care. Likelihood ratios use the sensitivity and specificity of a test to help clinicians determine decisions. Fortunately, you will most likely not need to calculate the sensitivity or specificity of common orthopedic assessments. Reviewing the search methods covered in chapter 2, take some time and look up the sensitivity and specificity of common orthopedic tests you use in your practice. You can use those values to calculate the likelihood ratios as we go through this section.

Likelihood ratios (LRs) are used to determine probability. Remember that no test is perfect, so there is no acceptable set of values, and your clinical decisions should be based on the potential implications of being wrong.[2,6] A positive LR (+LR) predicts positive pathology, and a negative LR (−LR) predicts that the injury is not present. Likelihood ratio values may range from 1,000 to 0.001, but a +LR greater than 5 and a −LR below 0.20 are believed to increase diagnostic confidence.[6] Table 3.1 provides details about the impact LRs have on probabilities.

Table 3.2 shows the calculated sensitivity and specificity values for the Lachman's test and pivot shift test of our athlete with the torn ACL. A +LR is calculated by dividing sensitivity by 1 minus specificity:

$$+LR = sensitivity / (1 - specificity)$$

It is the true positive rate corrected for the false positive rate.[6] The –LR is calculated by dividing 1 minus the sensitivity by the specificity:

$$(1 - sensitivity) / specificity$$

It is the false negative rate corrected for the true negative rate.[6] You would calculate a +LR when the test you are using depicts a positive result. In our sample data, the +LR for the Lachman's test is this:

$$0.80 / (1 - 0.89)$$

$$0.80 / 0.11 = 7.27$$

To explain this to an athlete, you would say that the positive Lachman's test indicates that she is 7.27 times more likely to have ruptured her ACL. Remember, though, that any +LR value between 5 and 10 will have only a moderate impact on your clinical decision. If you look back at figure 3.3, you will recall that in this sample data, the Lachman's test incorrectly depicted 100 ACL tears. To calculate the –LR for the Lachman's test in our sample data, you have this:

$$(1 - 0.8) / 0.89$$

$$0.2 / 0.89 = 0.22$$

You would calculate this if your Lachman's test was negative and depicted that the athlete did not have an ACL tear. In this case, you would tell your athlete that based on the negative Lachman's test, she most likely does not have a torn ACL. A

Table 3.1 Likelihood Ratio Impacts on Probabilities Postassessment

Positive likelihood ratio (+LR)		Negative likelihood ratio (–LR)	
Large impact	>10	Large impact	<0.1
Moderate impact	5 to 10	Moderate impact	0.1 to 0.2
Small impact	2 to 5	Small impact	0.2 to 0.5
Negligible impact	<2	Negligible impact	0.5 to 1.0

Data from J. Cleland, 2007, *Orthopaedic clinical examination: An evidence-based approach for physical therapists.* (Philadelphia, PA: Saunders).

Table 3.2 Likelihood Ratio Sample Calculations

	Lachman's test	Pivot shift test
Sensitivity	80%, or 0.8, for LR	90%, or 0.9, for LR
Specificity	89%, or 0.89, for LR	98.8%, or 0.988, for LR

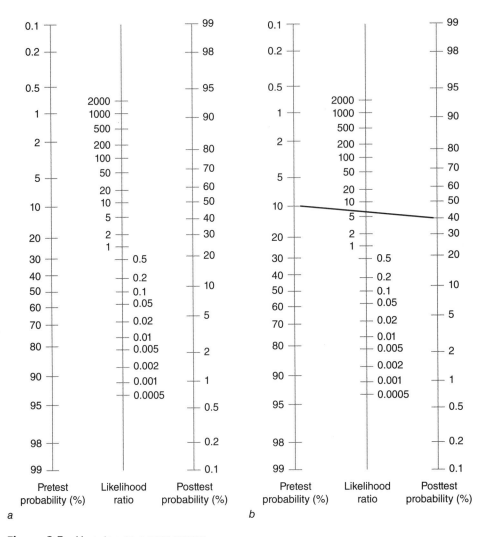

Figure 3.5 How to use a nomogram.

Adapted from Fagan TJ, Nomogram for Bayes theorem, *N Engl J Med.* 1975: 293:257, 1975.

value of 0.22 supports a small risk that the clinical decision is incorrect and would have a large impact on the probability and clinical decision. In our sample data, the Lachman's test is moderately strong at predicting a torn ACL when an ACL is torn, but this test could be better. However, if the Lachman's test is negative, it is robust in ruling out an ACL tear. Now using the values in table 3.2, calculate the +LR and –LR for the pivot shift test and decide what to tell your athlete in the event of a positive and a negative pivot shift test. The answers are in table 3.3.

The final tool to further assist you in making clinical decisions is a **nomogram** (figure 3.5*a*)—a graphic representation comparing pretest probability, the LRs, and posttest probability. Pretest probability is determined by the clinician based on history, signs and symptoms (S&S), and clinical experience. Returning to the athlete with the ACL tear, you believe that she has not torn her ACL because the S&S are not consistent, the athlete fails to report any sensations of giving way or

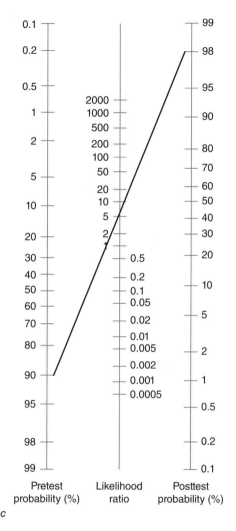

Figure 3.5 *(continued)*

Table 3.3 Likelihood Ratios for the Pivot Shift Test

+LR	75.0	Based on the positive pivot shift test, the athlete is 75 times more likely to have ruptured the ACL. Because this is a large impact, you would simply tell her that you believe that she has ruptured her ACL.
−LR	0.1	A negative pivot shift test supports that the athlete does not have a torn ACL.

instability, and there has been no effusion around the knee. Subsequently, you rate this athlete's pretest probability at 10%. Now, using a straightedge ruler, align one end of the ruler to the 10 on the pretest value line (figure 3.5*b*). Recalling that the +LR for the Lachman's test was 7, align the ruler so that it touches both the 10 on the Pretest Probability line and the 7 (approximate) on the Likelihood Ratio line. The right side of the ruler should now align with a value on the Posttest Probability line

Critical Appraisal of Evidence

In this critical appraisal of evidence, we are evaluating a few sections of a mock study that resembles what you might find in a literature review.

Study Overview

A pilot study to evaluate the effectiveness of ultrasound on perception of pain and relative improvement on various conditions that cause pain. All study participants had a history of multiple pain episodes and a history of rehabilitation therapies.

Methods

Three men and eight women ranging in age from 16 to 84 participated in the study. Each completed a visual analog pain scale (VAS) to rate pain from 0 to 10 (0 being no pain and 10 being severe pain) as intake scores. The treatment for each participant was the same except for the treatment area. The treatment was 3.3 MHz for 5 minutes at 1.5 W/cm^2 or 1 MHz for 5 minutes at 1.5 W/cm^2. Participants were also grouped based on chronicity of the condition, either acute (less than 8 weeks) or chronic (more than 8 weeks).

Results

The average intake score of the chronic group was 5.83, and the average exit score was 4.33, showing a measured improvement quotient of 25.7%. The average intake score of the acute group was 6.6, and the average exit score was 3.4, showing a measured improvement score of 48.5%.

Pain area	Diagnosis	Chronicity	Number of treatments
Wrist	Carpal tunnel syndrome	Chronic	5
Hip	Bursitis	Chronic	5
Ankle	Postsurgery	Chronic	7
Right foot	Fasciitis	Chronic	6
Knee	MCL sprain	Acute	4
Wrist	Carpal tunnel syndrome	Acute	6
Knee	Bursitis	Acute	3
Left elbow	Tendinitis	Acute	6
Both wrists	Hook of hamate	Acute	3
Neck	Cervical	Acute	7
Thumb	Degenerative joint disease	Acute	5

Critical Appraisal

1. The participants have a vast difference in age (16 to 84), and the sub-sequent results of treatments may vary substantially. When reviewing articles, you want to ensure that the populations are similar. You also want to ensure an equal and representative number of men and women.

2. The methods section fails to indicate whether the ultrasound was continuous or pulsed and whether thermal or nonthermal treatments were desired or conducted. Also, the authors stated that each treatment was the same except for the area of treatment, but then highlighted two treatment parameters.

3. The results highlight improvement scores but fail to state or show whether those scores are clinically significant or meaningful.

4. The table in the results section is inconsistent. The pain column fails to identify the left or right side of the body consistently. The diagnosis column is nondescript, and the number of treatments is inconsistent.

5. The reader is unable to determine which treatment was provided to each participant and whether the participant is male or female. Also not reported are any previous therapies participants may have had.

In conclusion, the clinician is unable to use any part of this research article to properly determine an appropriate course of treatment.

at approximately 45%. This means that based on a positive Lachman's test, there is a 45% chance of the athlete having a torn ACL.

Now let's assume that, as the clinician, you believe that the athlete has an ACL tear because she reports sensations of giving way, reports having been hit from behind below the knee, has significant knee effusion, and states that this injury feels strikingly similar to the ACL tear she had two years ago on the other knee. In this case, you feel 90% confident before you even perform the Lachman's test that the ACL is torn. Aligning the ruler with the 90 on the Pretest Probability line and the 7 on the Likelihood Ratio line, you see a posttest probability of 98% to 99% that this athlete has torn her ACL (figure 3.5c). The process is the same if you are using a +LR or a –LR, because the nomogram takes into account your impression. Remember that one of the primary aspects of evidence-based practice is your expertise, which is tied to research and athlete preference.

Summary

The goal of orthopedic assessments is to correctly classify athletes as injured or not injured. The objective is to protect the athlete and make an appropriate return-to-play decision, create a therapy plan, or make a referral. The goal is to make a competent clinical diagnosis in the absence of more invasive techniques such as arthroscopic surgery or to avoid unnecessary radiological exams and placing the athlete at risk for greater injury. This requires skill in coaching the athlete to be honest and forthcoming with signs and symptoms and in providing verbal cues and displaying confidence to help the athlete relax so you can administer an orthopedic exam. You also need significant experience to draw on in making choices and must remain vigilant in reviewing the current best practices and listening to the goals and concerns of the athlete. Beyond reviewing best practices, you must be able to interpret them so that you can apply them and improve athlete outcomes.

References

1. Rubin A, Bellamy J. *Practitioner's guide to using research for evidence-based practice.* 2nd ed. Hoboken, NJ: Wiley; 2012.

2. Fetters LK, Tilson J. *Evidence based physical therapy.* Philadelphia: Davis; 2012.

3. Broglio S, Ferrara M, Macciocchi S, Baumgartner T, Elliot R. Test-retest reliability of computerized concussion assessment programs. *Journal of Athletic Training.* 2007;42(4):509.

4. Hicks C. *Research methods for clinical therapists, applied project design and analysis.* 5th ed. New York: Churchill Livingstone; 2009.

5. Hemphill J. Interpreting the magnitudes of correlation coefficients. *American Psychologist.* 2003;58(1):78-80.

6. Di Fabio RP. *Essentials of rehabilitation research: A statistical guide to clinical practice.* Philadelphia: Davis; 2013.

7. Brenner H, Gefeller O. Variation of sensitivity, specificity, likelihood ratios and predictive values with disease prevalence. *Statistics in Medicine.* 1997;16:981-991.

8. Denegar C, Saliba E, Saliba S. *Therapeutic modalities for musculoskeletal injuries.* 3rd ed. Champaign, IL: Human Kinetics; 2010.

9. Clinically Relevant Technologies. Clinical orthopedic exam (CORE). [Mobile application software]. www.clinicallyrelevant.com. 2012.

10. Kanchanaraksa S. Evaluation of diagnostic and screening tests: Validity and reliability. http://ocw.jhsph.edu/courses/fundepi/PDFs/Lecture11.pdf. Accessed March 20, 2014.

PART II

Critical Appraisal of Evidence-Based Practice

Part II takes you through the types of evidence you may seek during your EBP searches. However, not all evidence is created equal. Further, not all journals require the same rigor of review before a study is published. Therefore, you must be able to critically appraise the research studies you find. Although this may sound like an intimidating task, we take you step by step through a critical appraisal outline in each chapter and provide examples along the way.

Chapter 4 describes diagnostic research. These types of studies are of techniques that help clinicians diagnose injuries or illnesses. Chapter 5 addresses prognostic research, which involves the study of techniques that help clinicians with treatment and rehabilitation decisions once the injury or illness is diagnosed. Both of these chapters present exercises that teach you how to locate these types of research articles. Each chapter ends with a section on how to perform a critical appraisal of that type of research article, complete with a step-by-step process that you can use long into the future.

Chapter 6 introduces systematic reviews, meta-analyses, and critically appraised topics. These types of studies look at multiple independent research articles on the same topic, evaluate each article using several metrics, and then provide a summary of the findings on that topic based on the combined outcomes of the independent studies. These types of research studies represent the highest levels of evidence and are at the very top of the evidence pyramid. Chapter 6 also provides strategies for finding these types of studies and offers the opportunity to practice a search.

Chapter 7 takes all of the information presented earlier in the text and discusses how to put it to use in your daily clinical practice. Examples of how to balance the evidence you find with your own clinical expertise and your athletes' values are presented. Communication is key. Additionally, other resources are discussed, such as clinical practice guideline databases, RSS feeds, and suggestions for practicing altruism with the provision of health care for your athletes.

Chapter 8 provides an overview of outcome measures that are emerging in the field of health care. Many of these involve the athlete's level of satisfaction or perceived improvements, including quality of life measures. The chapter also explains how to use the outcomes once you find the high-quality evidence you're looking for. What happens after you implement the new evidence into your practice? How can you tell whether your athletes are benefiting (which is the ultimate concern)? The chapter concludes with strategies for adjusting your practice based on your outcomes.

With the critical appraisal concepts, outlines, and practices presented in part II, you will be ready to begin transforming your daily practice to provide high-quality care to your athletes based on the most current evidence.

CHAPTER 4

Diagnostic Research

Objectives

After reading this chapter, you will be able to do the following:

- Assess the quality of an article regarding the clarity of the definition of the measurement of interest.
- Determine whether the researcher has adequate methods to measure the data.
- Tell whether a study population is clearly defined.
- Recognize whether the researcher protects against bias and maximizes reliability.
- Determine whether the article meaningfully relates to your athlete.

The process of diagnostic research begins by defining what a researcher aims to analyze. Often this is a disease, disorder, or injury that would be common in athletic training. The researcher must clearly define what will be measured. Assuming it is the **quantifiable** laxity of an ACL, the researcher must have adequate methods of measuring that laxity beyond simple **subjective** assessments. The researcher then develops a plan to safeguard against bias or causes of unreliability and selects a representative sample of participants. The study design should ensure the efficient use of participants' time and maximize reliable data collection. Collected data are analyzed using a variety of methods and then presented for review and publication. As an evidence-based clinician, you must then determine whether all of the preceding was accomplished and whether the study will assist you in assessing or providing care to your own athletes. This chapter will help you assess the methods in a study, determine whether the population is clearly defined, and identify any risks of bias.

Measurement

Let's first look at the value of diagnostic tests in athletic training. The perfect test would unequivocally identify the presence or absence of a condition. We know from previous chapters and experience that noninvasive assessments alone are not perfect predictors without additional information (e.g., a history, signs and symptoms, multiple tests). Measurements performed during diagnostic tests should be reproducible, accurate, and feasible. A feasible test would be rapid, easy to perform, cost effective, and harmless. Prior to selecting a diagnostic test, you should ask yourself the following questions: What information do I need? Will this test support or fail to support my clinical hypothesis? Will this test influence the treatments I select for my athlete?[1]

Answering these questions will require you to follow the steps of performing a literature search outlined in chapter 2. What exactly do you want to search for? What type of research study or publication will help you answer your questions? In general, you want to know how reproducible a test is, how accurate it is, how the test results will affect your decision, what the costs and risk of the test are, and whether performing the test will improve the clinical outcome or have an adverse effect. Some tests might carry risks or have serious consequences (e.g., an apprehension test could cause shoulder dislocations; CAT scans increase the risk for cancer; a patellar subluxation test can cause subluxation). Unless you are sure the test is necessary, it might not be worth the risk.

True Agreement Versus Chance

To assess the reproducibility of a test, search for studies looking at the test's intra- and interrater reliability. Remember that intrarater reliability refers to agreement among repeated assessments of the test by the same person. Interrater reliability refers to agreement across repeated assessments of a test by more than one person. There will be some degree of variability between these repeated assessments, but the statistical report should involve proportion agreement, or **Cohen's kappa**. With kappa, which is reported as κ (similar to correlations and *r* mentioned in chapter 3), a score of 1 is complete agreement and a score of 0 is no agreement. The benefit of reporting κ over *r* is that it measures true agreement over chance agreement between raters. A simple correlation between two rates or assessors provides an *r* value. However, a correlation between raters or ratings may occur merely by chance, which would not be true agreement. Kappa is more robust in that it takes into account both the observed agreement and a proportion of agreement that can be expected to occur by chance.[2]

At this point you have established that a test has an acceptable measure of reproducibility, but this does not mean that it actually measures what you want. It simply means that you are getting the same result, a result that may or may not be accurate. You now want to determine the accuracy of the test.

Test Accuracy

A **cross-sectional study** assesses a population on the presence of an illness or condition by comparing a new assessment with a gold standard assessment. A **case control study** is performed in the same way but is carried out on a sample of people with an injury or illness. Again, the gold standard test to detect the condition is compared to a more novel method of assessment. The relation between the gold standard test and the novel assessment is recorded in terms of sensitivity, specificity, or likelihood ratios.

Sensitivity and specificity are good at separating a very sick person and a very healthy person. They help to differentiate between an absolute injury and the absence of an injury. However, what if an athlete is not fully healthy but not very sick? What if the ACL is only partially torn? These questions highlight the weaknesses of diagnostic tests: they may not be that useful in identifying mild cases of disease or injury.

Recall the discussion in chapter 3 of false positive and false negative test results. A false positive is when a test shows the presence of a condition when it's not really present; this must be avoided to prevent unnecessary treatments or surgery. A false negative is when a test suggests that no injury is present, but one truly is; this can result in no treatment or no surgery being provided when it is needed.

To avoid these errors, researchers use **receiver operating characteristic (ROC) curves**. ROC curves are a graphic representation of sensitivity and specificity, with sensitivity on the vertical axis and the value of 1 – specificity on the horizontal axis. Figure 4.1 displays three curves representing worthless, good, and excellent prediction examples. Accuracy is represented by the area under the curve; the greater the area under the curve is, the more accurate the test is. In a dichotomous situation in which athletes are already clearly classified as having or not having a condition, the test in question is performed on those with the condition. An abnormal test, or one detecting disease, falls under the curve. The exact calculations for developing an ROC curve are not important, but it is important to understand that the closer a prediction method or test is to real-world scenarios, the closer a coordinate point at the top left corner of the graph will appear.

Figure 4.2 depicts a hypothetical ROC curve analysis of predicting ACL tears based on two clinical factors. Hormone variation is a predictor, but adding a Q-angle measurement improves the ability to predict an ACL tear.

Retrospective and Prospective Studies

A clinical decision based on evidence requires understanding the published reproducibility and accuracy of tests used in the profession of athletic training.

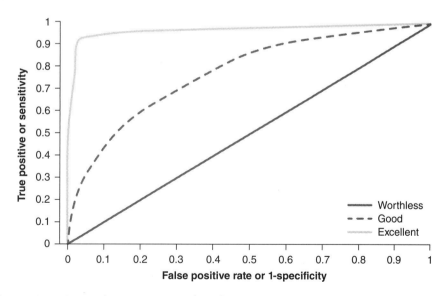

Figure 4.1 Comparing ROC curve values for meaning.

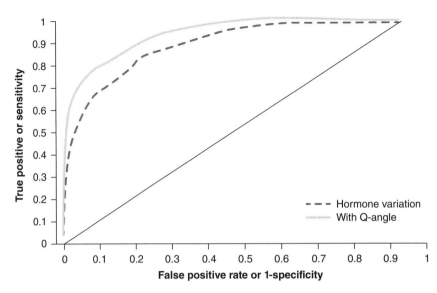

Figure 4.2 Hypothetical prediction of ACL tear risk.

However, it's also important to review retrospective studies and follow prospective studies. A **prospective study** follows a group of similar people (e.g., athletes) over a period of time to determine whether certain factors or conditions affect future injury prevalence. Athletic trainers use this type of knowledge to prevent injury. An example would be following a group of athletes who have had Tommy John surgeries using a new technique. To assess the costs, risks, and acceptability of a new surgical procedure, we need to have long-term follow-up. If a new surgical procedure results in 25% of athletes needing a revision upon returning to sport, compared to only 11% needing a revision after the traditional technique, doctors will stop performing the new technique. Likewise, if return to sport after a new surgical technique is two or three months sooner than after a traditional technique, it may be beneficial to continue using it. The greater the number of events (revisions needed or faster return to sport), the greater our confidence in making a decision.

A **retrospective study** is similar to a prospective study, except that researchers look back at the histories of similar groups; it's a historical review. A large majority of concussion research is retrospective. We are currently reviewing historical data of similar athletes (e.g., American football players, soccer players, and boxers) and realizing the long-term effects of repeated head trauma. Retrospective studies are excellent resources to help athletic trainers prevent injury and illness.

Risks

The final consideration related to testing and assessment is the impact of the test on the athlete. Is there a risk in performing the diagnostic test? Might the test itself affect future testing? Let's look at the risk involved in certain types of tests. Consider an athlete who has signs and symptoms of allergies. You, the parents, and a team physician agree that the athlete should undergo allergy testing. Although generally safe and involving small amounts of allergens, an allergy test involves repeated skin punctures and thus a risk of causing allergic reactions or infection (or both). Immediate rashes and hives might be treated with Benadryl; however, if the athlete has never been treated with certain medications, a severe reaction can occur.

When an athlete suffers head trauma, an attending physician may need to decide whether to perform an X-ray, MRI, or CAT scan. The physician considers the long-term increased cancer risk due to exposure to the CAT scan and the lesser cancer risk of an X-ray or MRI. These are direct impacts on physical health, but cognitive tests also affect athletes. Repeating a cognitive assessment to assess mental capacity or function might result in the athlete's learning methods to improve her testing scores. Psychometric test properties of popular concussion assessment programs for athletes without concussions range in sensitivity from 9.3 to 93%; specificity values range from 78.8 to 95.2%. This indicates less-than-optimal reliability, or the ability of these tests to predict concussion or recovery. Pearson's r and the intraclass correlation coefficient (ICC) are frequently used to report reliability between test and retest results.[2] In the case of psychometric testing, r values range from .30 and .88, and ICC values range from .15 to .87.[2] This reveals some level of inconsistency between test sessions; thus, no single cognitive test should serve as a return-to-play tool.

Methods

Chapter 1 outlined the following five steps of evidence-based practice:

1. Create a clinically relevant and searchable question concerning your athlete.
2. Conduct a database search to find the best evidence.
3. Critically appraise the articles or evidence for quality.
4. Critically synthesize the evidence to choose and implement a treatment.
5. Assess the outcomes by monitoring the athlete.

Chapter 2 demonstrated how to perform a database search, and chapter 3 introduced ways to understand and evaluate the evidence. This chapter continues the discussion of evaluation methods by addressing how to appraise the diagnostic articles you have found. Following are four steps to appraising diagnostic research:[1]

1. Determine the applicability to your athlete.
2. Assess the quality of the article.
3. Review the results.
4. Summarize the clinical bottom line.

As you gather your articles using a variety of search methods, you can apply a simple assessment to quickly and easily eliminate low-quality articles. Review any article based on the following five criteria (CRAAP):

- **Currency:** Is it current, or generally published in the last 10 years or so depending on the likelihood that the information has been updated?
- **Relevance:** Does the title of the article relate to your topic or needs?
- **Authority:** Are the authors qualified to publish on the topic?

Foundations of Evidence:
Steps to Appraising Diagnostic Research

1. Determine the applicability to your athlete.
2. Assess the quality of the article.
3. Review the results.
4. Summarize the clinical bottom line.

- **Accuracy:** Is the source reliable and truthful?
- **Purpose:** Is the purpose of the publication to inform, teach, sell, entertain, or persuade?

See the sidebar CRAAP Criteria for Evaluating Published Articles for detailed questions to ask to preliminarily assess articles.

- **Currency.** Is the information in need of being revised? The 2004 National Athletic Trainers' Association (NATA) position statement on the management of sport-related concussion allowed for same-day return to participation if symptoms resolved and the athlete passed a return-to-play test.[3] The 2014 position statement update noted that our knowledge about how to treat concussions had significantly changed and ruled guidelines as recent as 10 years old obsolete.

- **Relevance.** Is the article written at a level appropriate for your needs, and do you understand it? If not, you may fail to reach a valid conclusion about the use of assessments in your situation. Has the information been peer reviewed, or is it an editorial or opinion piece? Editorials often have a bias and lack the scientific rigor required to make the information useful for sound clinical decisions.

- **Authority.** Is a sponsor involved that has a product to market? If so, read the information with great care. If an article is promoting an aquatics rehab program to aid in the recovery of knee surgery, but it was sponsored by a company that sells therapy pools, you need to suspect some potential bias. These types of conflicts of interest can be questionable.

- **Accuracy.** After completing your primary review, it is time to dig a little deeper and appraise the article. The Quality Assessment of Diagnostic Accuracy Studies (QUADAS) is a 14-question instrument to assist you in the appraisal (see the sidebar).[1,4] The answer choices are *yes, no,* or *uncertain*; a greater number of *yes* answers is preferred.[1] There is no set number of acceptable *yes* answers, but if any *uncertain* or *no* answers make you feel uncomfortable using the data to make a clinical decision, you may want to further research the topic and expand the number of articles you review.

- **Purpose.** Why is the information presented? Is it an advertisement? Is it funded by someone with a financial stake in selling something? If the answer to the preceding questions is yes, be sure to thoroughly review the academic content. The purpose of a quality article is to inform and provide outcomes, allowing readers to apply it as they see fit.

CRAAP Criteria for Evaluating Published Articles

Currency: The timeliness of the information
- When was the information published or posted?
- Has the information been revised or updated?
- Does your topic require current information, or will older sources work as well?

Relevance: The importance of the information for your needs
- Does the information relate to your topic or answer your question?
- Who is the intended audience?
- Is the information at an appropriate level (i.e., not too elementary or advanced for your needs)?
- Have you looked at a variety of sources?

Authority: The source of the information
- Who is the author, publisher, source, or sponsor?
- What are the author's credentials or organizational affiliations?
- Is the author qualified to write on the topic?

Accuracy: The reliability, truthfulness, and correctness of the content
- Where does the information come from?
- Is the information supported by evidence?
- Has the information been reviewed or refereed?
- Can you verify any of the information in another source or from personal knowledge?
- Does the language or tone seem unbiased and free of emotion?

Purpose: The reason the information exists
- What is the purpose of the information? Is it to inform, teach, sell, entertain, or persuade?
- Do the authors or sponsors make their intentions or purpose clear?
- Is the information fact, opinion, or propaganda?
- Does the point of view appear objective and impartial?
- Are there political, ideological, cultural, religious, institutional, or personal biases?

Adapted, by permission, librarians at CSU Chico, 2014, *The CRAAP test - evaluating web resources* (Chico, CA: California State University). Available: http://libguides.library.ncat.edu/content.php?pid = 53820&sid = 394505. Accessed 6/1/2014, 2014.

Using the Quality Assessment of Diagnostic Accuracy Studies to Assess Diagnostic Articles

Answer each question as *yes, no,* or *uncertain.*

_____ 1. Was the spectrum of athletes representative of the athletes who will receive the test in practice?

_____ 2. Were selection criteria clearly described?

_____ 3. Is the reference standard likely to correctly classify the target condition?

_____ 4. Is the time period between reference standard and index test short enough to be reasonably sure that the target condition did not change between the two tests?

_____ 5. Did the whole sample or a random selection of the sample receive verification using a reference standard of diagnosis?

_____ 6. Did athletes receive the same reference standard regardless of the index test result?

_____ 7. Was the reference standard independent of the index test (i.e., the index test did not form part of the reference standard)?

_____ 8. Was the execution of the index test described in sufficient detail to permit replication of the test?

_____ 9. Was the execution of the reference standard described in sufficient detail to permit its replication?

_____ 10. Were the index test results interpreted without knowledge of the results of the reference standard?

_____ 11. Were the reference standard results interpreted without knowledge of the results of the index test?

_____ 12. Were the same clinical data available when test results were interpreted as would be available when the test is used in practice?

_____ 13. Were uninterpretable or intermediate test results reported?

_____ 14. Were withdrawals from the study explained?

Reprinted from P.F. Whiting et al., 2006, "Evaluation of QUADAS, a tool for the quality assessment of diagnostic accuracy studies," *BMC Medical Research Methodology* 6: 6:9. © BioMed Central Ltd.

Each of the questions should be clearly addressed or answered in the article. If you are interested in learning whether a rehab program would be appropriate for high school athletes, the studies you review should have been conducted with people in the same age range. This is called generalizability—that is, can the results of a study be applied to another population based on similarities in the populations?

Authors should clearly tell you how they selected participants and why, as well as any reasons participants were excluded from participation. Did the author report issues with the data that could not be explained, and was the number of participants at the start and end of the study reported? If fewer completed the study than initiated it, was there an explanation for the dropout rate? If an author was researching the use of latex bandages to decrease swelling after ankle sprains and a volunteer participant had an allergy to latex, that person would need to leave the study. In this case, an author should report that 40 subjects volunteered to participate and were initially taking part in the study, and one was removed because of an exclusionary criterion. The author should not say that 39 people agreed to participate.

Similarly, if a new test (index test) is being assessed, it should be compared to an appropriate gold standard reference. If a researcher is testing a new axillary thermometer to establish whether it accurately assesses core body temperature, it should be compared to rectal thermometer measures. Comparing a new axillary thermometer to oral thermometers or others that are not scientifically accepted as the gold standard could introduce significant error, which would make the study results inappropriate to use in clinical practice.

Also important when appraising an article is assessing its methods section. Is it detailed enough that you could replicate it, if desired? You should be able to fully understand what was done during the study when reading the methods section.

The prevention of bias is also important during a study. If a participant was assessed using both an indexed and a referenced test, were the results interpreted separately? In other words, did the person completing the assessments know the results of the comparative assessment? A person who is aware of the other outcomes when completing an assessment creates a potential for biased reporting and a loss of objectivity, which is important in research.

Consider a scenario in which you are the athletic trainer at a school, and a number of female soccer players have had neck injuries. These injuries are secondary to being hit in the head with a soccer ball or falling and trying to keep the head from striking the ground. You perform an evidence-based search using the CINAHL, Cochrane, Medline, and PubMed databases with the search terms *neck, injury,* and *female.* One of the articles you retrieve is titled "Extension Neck Injury in Female DanceSport Competitors" in the *International Journal of Athletic Training and Therapy* (McCrabe, 2014). See the Critical Appraisal of Evidence sidebar for more on this study.

Changing the scenario, you now have a group of postconcussion high school athletes, and you are in need of quantifiable methods to assess their balance. Again, you perform an evidence-based search using the CINAHL, Cochrane, Medline, and PubMed databases using the search terms *postural, balance, BESS,* and *scoring.* One of the articles you retrieve is titled "Comparison of a Mobile Technology Application With the Balance Error Scoring System" (see figure 4.3 for a screenshot of this article's abstract).

Critical Appraisal of Evidence

In this critical appraisal of evidence, we are evaluating the global context of the following article in a preliminary manner:

McCrabe TR, Ambegaonkar JP, Wyon M, Redding E. Extension neck injury in female DanceSport competitors. *IJATT*. 2014; 19 (3): 19, 32-36.

Study Overview

This study assesses the extension neck injury (ENI) of dancers. ENI is not well understood, but it occurs when a ballroom dancer is required to hold her head in extension and rotated left during a dance.

Methods

The study uses a 42-question electronic survey to assess the prevalence of ENI in ballroom dancers. The survey used drop-down, multiple-choice, and short-answer questions. It was distributed to 127 ballroom dancers via e-mail and social networking, and 87 completed the survey.

Critical Appraisal

You are unfamiliar with the demands of DanceSport, so you start with the CRAAP test for a preliminary review.

1. *Is this article current?* Yes, it was published in 2014.
2. *Is it relevant?* No, the context of the article does not appear to relate to the contact and falling injuries that your players are experiencing. This article relates to holding a neck position for a period of time.
3. Having determined that this article is not relevant, you can discard it and continue your review of other articles. This is an example of a preliminary review.

Your preliminary review reveals that the article is indeed current and relevant and has a qualified author. The information appears accurate, and the purpose is to inform clinicians about an alternative to the BESS test. You are now going to read the article and use the QUADAS to assess it, answering each question *yes*, *no*, or *uncertain*. After completing your assessment, compare it to the following sample interpretation and explanation.

- Item 1, No. You are looking at high school athletes, and this study uses non-athletic college students.
- Item 2, No. You are told who the participants are, but not why they were selected. They may have been students in a class, they may have been paid, or they may have been recruited leaving a movie theater or a skating rink. These variables could influence their ability to balance or their desire to perform during the study.

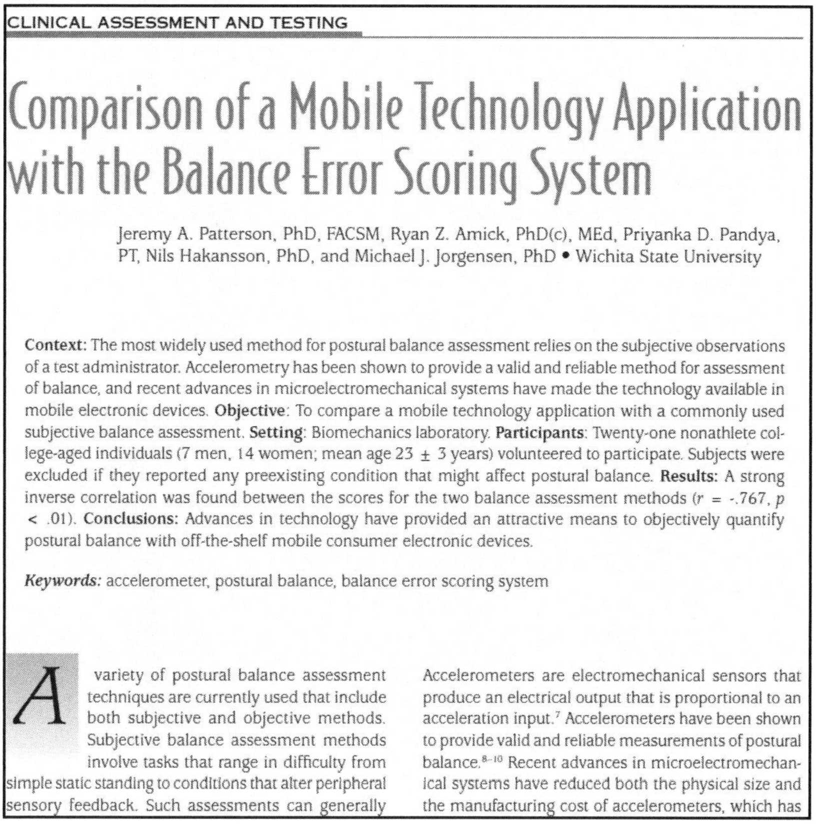

CLINICAL ASSESSMENT AND TESTING

Comparison of a Mobile Technology Application with the Balance Error Scoring System

Jeremy A. Patterson, PhD, FACSM, Ryan Z. Amick, PhD(c), MEd, Priyanka D. Pandya, PT, Nils Hakansson, PhD, and Michael J. Jorgensen, PhD ▪ Wichita State University

Context: The most widely used method for postural balance assessment relies on the subjective observations of a test administrator. Accelerometry has been shown to provide a valid and reliable method for assessment of balance, and recent advances in microelectromechanical systems have made the technology available in mobile electronic devices. **Objective**: To compare a mobile technology application with a commonly used subjective balance assessment. **Setting**: Biomechanics laboratory. **Participants**: Twenty-one nonathlete college-aged individuals (7 men, 14 women; mean age 23 ± 3 years) volunteered to participate. Subjects were excluded if they reported any preexisting condition that might affect postural balance. **Results:** A strong inverse correlation was found between the scores for the two balance assessment methods ($r = -.767$, $p < .01$). **Conclusions:** Advances in technology have provided an attractive means to objectively quantify postural balance with off-the-shelf mobile consumer electronic devices.

Keywords: accelerometer, postural balance, balance error scoring system

A variety of postural balance assessment techniques are currently used that include both subjective and objective methods. Subjective balance assessment methods involve tasks that range in difficulty from simple static standing to conditions that alter peripheral sensory feedback. Such assessments can generally Accelerometers are electromechanical sensors that produce an electrical output that is proportional to an acceleration input.[7] Accelerometers have been shown to provide valid and reliable measurements of postural balance.[8-10] Recent advances in microelectromechanical systems have reduced both the physical size and the manufacturing cost of accelerometers, which has

Figure 4.3 Abstract of article "Comparison of a Mobile Technology Application With the Balance Error Scoring System."

Reprinted from J.A. Patterson et al., 2014, "Comparison of a mobile technology application with the balance error scoring system," *International Journal of Athletic Therapy & Training* 19: 4-7.

- Item 3, No. In this case, the referenced standard is the BESS test. The author reports that the BESS test has moderate to good reliability but that values have varied greatly. This fails to support the notion that the BESS test may indeed correctly identify your athletes with or without balance problems secondary to their concussions. The author also mentions that the BESS test was modified to replicate the holding of the iPad to the chest instead of having the hands on the hips. Any alteration in a reference test invalidates the previously established reliability values for the test. A more robust or gold standard test to use as the reference would have been technologies that use a force plate to measure instability.

- Item 4, Uncertain. It can be assumed that the two tests were performed one after the other, but the author does not mention an exact time frame between assessments. Too short a period could lead to fatigue during the second test and increase error into the results.

- Item 5, Yes. The entire sample was assessed with the same reference test (BESS).

- Item 6, Yes.

- Item 7, No. The reference test was modified to be similar to the index test.
- Items 8 and 9, No. The length of the test is unknown, and the directions provided are also not indicated. The author states that assessments took place on a solid support surface and on compliant foam. The exact type of solid surface is not revealed (e.g., carpet, tile, wood). There is also no description of the density or thickness of the compliant foam. The participant in the picture is wearing shoes. Did all participants wear shoes? Did the shoes vary in thickness? If so, that would introduce error to the results.
- Items 10 and 11, Uncertain. The author fails to indicate whether the researchers were aware of the scores on one assessment when scoring the other. The author also reports the average BESS scores between the raters but fails to report the interrater reliability.
- Item 12, Yes. It is safe to assume that in practice the athletic trainer could measure weight and height, calculate BMI, and request the age of the subjects.
- Item 13, No. The author did not directly mention any uninterpretable results.
- Item 14, No. The author did not state the initial enrollment number or final number that would indicate any withdrawals.

Upon completion of the QUADAS and a detailed review of the article, you see that the study has numerous weaknesses. You may not be able to use the methods in this study at your high school to assess balance in athletes postconcussion.

Foundations of Evidence: Appraising Diagnostic Studies

Question	Location in the article
Is my athlete represented in this sample?	Methods
Are the tests used in the study accurate?	Background, Methods, Results
Was the novel or index test compared to a gold standard assessment?	Methods
Were tests performed by skilled clinicians, and were they blinded to the results of the other test?	Methods
Were participants exposed to both the index and the reference test?	Methods
Were useful statistics reported and usable for clinical application?	Results
Will the test outcomes help me treat my athlete?	Discussion

Adapted from Fetters and Tilson 2012.

Summary

The primary purpose of learning how to critically appraise research is to make you an educated consumer of knowledge so you can practice as an evidence-based clinician. The main goal of evidence-based practice is to ensure that you provide the absolute best care to athletes. Learning to review the steps of a preliminary assessment and a detailed assessment decreases the chances that you use an assessment that is not suited for the situation. It enables you to question the methods, results, and discussions and not simply accept whatever is published as absolute truth. Balancing your gut feelings that come from clinical experience, the use of accurate research, and input from your athletes will lead to improved outcomes and create an evidence-based practice.

References

1. Fetters LK, Tilson J. *Evidence based physical therapy*. Philadelphia: Davis; 2012.

2. Vaz S, Falkmer T, Passmore A, Parsons R, Andreou P. The case for using the repeatability coefficient when calculating test retest reliability. *PLOS ONE*. 2013;8(9):1-7.

3. Guskiewicz K, Bruce S, Cantu R, et al. National athletic trainers' association position statement: Management of sport-related concussion. *JAT*. 2004;39(3):280-297.

4. Whiting PF, Weswood ME, Rutjes AWS, Reitsma JB, Bossuyt PNM, Kleijnen J. Evaluation of QUADAS, a tool for the quality assessment of diagnostic accuracy studies. *BMC Medical Research Methodology*. 2006;6:9-8.

CHAPTER 5

Prognostic Research

Objectives

After reading this chapter, you will be able to do the following:

- Explain the prognostic appraisal process.
- Assess prognostic studies for validity.
- Interpret results of prognostic studies.

Prognosis is a principal component of athletic training. All athletic trainers have at some point in their careers had to answer questions such as these: Will this help me return to playing sooner? When will I be able to return to practice? How much longer will it be before I can run? These are all prognostic questions; the athletic trainer is being requested to forecast, or predict, an outcome. Prognostic research is different from diagnostic research. In the diagnostic process discussed in chapter 4, you used a method to assess an illness or injury and had to make a clinical decision based on your assessment. In prognostic situations, you already know the illness or injury and need to predict how long recovery will take or whether full recovery can be expected. Because often no specific tests to answer these questions exist, evidence-based clinicians use their best judgment based on their experience and review **prognostic research** to help them inform the athlete. When predicting the course of an illness or condition, it's important to take into account the athlete's age, sex, history, and symptoms and the results of other tests performed.[1] Remember that prognosis is not limited to athletes with a current illness or injury. You can often assess BMI, resting heart rate, sickle cell trait, or other factors to predict problems going forward. This chapter provides information to improve your prognostic abilities.

Prognostic Designs

Athletes vary in many ways, including size, strength, history, health, and sex, which complicates the development of a prognosis. Athletic trainers implicitly use many of these predictor characteristics to estimate an athlete's prognosis. Because prognostic studies lack controls, unlike diagnostic studies, it is wise to use a multivariable approach in the design and analysis of prognostic research. The athlete's outcome is often reported as a probability or risk based on prognostic models of research.

Common terms for prognostic models used in the literature include *prediction rules, prediction models,* and *risk scores.*[1]

The goal of prognostic research is to forecast outcomes based on a combination of predictors in a specific population. Participant predictors are obtained from the athlete's demographics, history, physical exam, and injury characteristics; the results from diagnostic tests; and any previous treatments and responses to those treatments. The impact of these in many circumstances are important but may be overshadowed by the variables of sex and age because the incidence of certain injuries varies by sex and age.[1] A female soccer player with a large Q angle may cause you more concern about ACL injury than a male with a similar issue, based on sex.

Any predictor variables used and reported in a prognostic study need to be clearly defined and reproducible. Cohort and case control studies are best for answering prognostic research questions. **Cohort studies** are prospective; they group subjects together over long periods of time to see whether they experience certain outcomes.[1,2] The outcome may be the resolution of a condition or the development of a new condition or injury. Prospective studies may be initiated at the start of an athletic season. An example is the assessment of knee ligament laxity, quadriceps strength compared to hamstring strength, and lower-extremity range of motion in a cohort of female volleyball players at class AAA high schools in Arizona to track the incidence of overuse knee injuries. At the end of the year, you would look for values in the baseline variables that may have attributed to the overuse conditions developed during the season. This sets the stage for establishing measures to prevent or decrease the prevalence of overuse injuries.

Retrospective case control studies are often used for prognostic analysis secondary to an observed pattern of injury. Although case control studies are valuable and noted extensively in the literature, they often have fewer controls on the data because they lack precise measurements. A retrospective study may be initiated after a districtwide insurance report depicts an increase in ankle sprains among football players from 32 in 2012 to 97 in 2013. The players are all returning players from the previous year at various high schools, are male, are of similar ages, and have similar playing experience. Although the research lacks anthropometric data or medical history information, the researchers can question what changed over the last year. In this example, let's assume that the new high schools switched from natural turf to a deep-padded artificial turf. The resulting action would be the same as that of a prospective cohort study: developing methods to prevent injuries.

Prognostic Statistics

The common statistics you will see reported in prognostic research studies are correlational, various types of regression, and ROC curves.

Correlation

A **correlation** is simply the degree to which two variables are related. It's important to remember that relationship is not causal; a change in one variable doesn't necessarily result in a change in another. For example, figure 5.1 shows a positive relationship between weight and height. As weight increases, so does height; this is an example of a positive correlation. Although this is typical, an increase in weight doesn't cause someone to become taller. Thus, these two variables are closely related, but one does not cause the other. It is very possible for a person to reach a height of 70 inches (178 cm) at a healthy 170 pounds (77 kg) but continue to gain weight. Other examples are age and the number of medical conditions experienced, and high SAT scores and high grades. Some very young people can have many medical conditions, and some students can perform well on the SAT but fail at school.

Recall from previous chapters that the closer a correlation is to the absolute value of 1, the stronger the relationship is (r varies between –1.0 and +1.0). A negative correlation might be explained using age and flexibility. As we age, we become less flexible, but being less flexible doesn't make us older (figure 5.2).

Although weight–height and age–flexibility are easy correlations to visualize (they would be near +1.0 and –1.0, respectively), other correlations in athletic training might be less easy to visualize, such as the correlation between the decrease in pain and swelling or the correlation between an increase in body mass and an increase in strength. Correlations are evaluated by how strongly one variable relates to another (table 5.1). In the literature you may find an r value recorded like this: r = .45, p < .05, in which p is the probability. In its most basic form, the p value is simply a probability that something could occur by chance alone.[3] We want to rule out the possibility of things happening by chance alone so we can say that a test or outcome

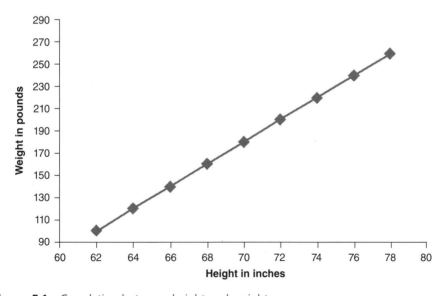

Figure 5.1   Correlation between height and weight.

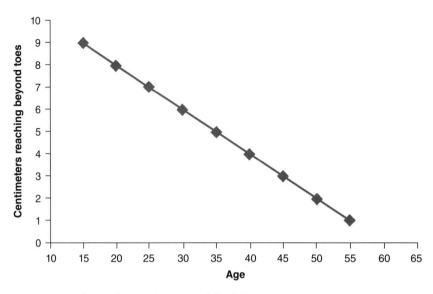

Figure 5.2 Correlation between age and flexibility.

Table 5.1 Correlation of Strength

Absolute value of r	Strength
.00–.25	Weak or no correlation
.26–.49	Low relationship
.50–.69	Moderate relationship
.70–.89	High relationship
.90–1.0	Very high relationship

is truly reliable. This means that we want small p values of .05 or .01. A value of .05 means that there is a 5% chance that the outcome occurred by chance alone; in other words, if we repeated the study 100 times, we should find the same result 95 times. Likewise, a p value of .01 is more exact and suggests that if the study were repeated 100 times, the outcome would be the same 99 times.

It's important to understand that the values of r and p are independent of each other. Let's assume that while reviewing an article, you see $r = .55, p < .01$. What does this mean? Reviewing table 5.1, you see that .55 is a moderate relationship and the significance is high. There is better than a 99% chance that you would find the same result if you repeated this study 100 times. To determine whether this is clinically significant, you would need to evaluate additional variables. Now, let's say you find $r = .09, p = .05$. The first thing to note is that there is no true strength in this correlation even though you have an acceptable p value indicating test reproducibility 95 out of 100 times. This should be interpreted as a reliable measure of two items that are truly not correlated. However, seeing an example of $r = .91, p = .78$, you may get excited to see a strong relationship between variables, but with a probability that says you would find that again only 22 out of 100 times, it's not reliable. Knowing how to calculate these values to appraise research is not important, but knowing what they mean is valuable.

One item that will vastly affect probability values is the number of participants. In studies with very large numbers of participants, many results might be significant; however, with a low r value, they might not be meaningful. Conversely, small sample sizes often have poor probability scores and may have high or very high relationship values. This is simply a result of the mathematical equations and supports why we often want to appraise studies with great numbers of subjects.

Regression

The second most common type of statistical test used during prognostic research is regression. **Regression** builds on multiple sets of correlational factors and samples where they overlap to make predictions. The symbol R^2 represents the results of a regression or prognostic equation. Similar to r used in correlation, the closer the value is to 1, the greater the predictive value is. Regression is almost intuitive if you think about the daily operations in an athletic training setting prior to a practice. As an athletic trainer, you informally assess numerous factors in predicting the risk of heat injury. This deduction is based on predictive variables: humidity, heat, wind speed, cloud cover, and an athlete's hydration and body composition as well as a history of having experienced heat illness. If the wind is still, there is no cloud cover, the humidity is 87% with an ambient temperature of 107 °F (41.7 °C) in the shade, and you have a football player with a BMI of 41 who is dehydrated according to a specific gravity assessment and he has previous experienced heat exhaustion, you can be pretty sure that this athlete is at risk during today's practice. Although this is a simple, straightforward example of regression, the same process is used in research studies. Regression is a complex equation that formally accounts for what we often do intuitively on samples and variables too complex to assess by hand. Although no single factor might result in a heat illness, the more contributing factors that are present, the more likely it is.

A Venn diagram is a simple illustrative method to demonstrate relations between variables. Figure 5.3 displays a simple Venn diagram. Each circle can be thought of as a pie chart or a complete percentage. Section A indicates the relationship between the Q angle and the risk of ACL rupture; the overlapping area is the percentage of ACL ruptures that can be contributed to Q-angle measures. Section B displays the percentage of ACL ruptures that can be attributed to hamstring weakness. The greater the overlap is, the stronger the relationship or potential contribution to a condition is. Section C shows that Q angle and hamstring weakness contribute to almost 50% of ACL ruptures. When predicting using regression, the more contributing variables you assess that are correlated with the variable of interest, the greater the chance is that you can predict the occurrence of a condition.

Appraisal Questions

When appraising prognostic research, you will use a process similar to the QUADAS from chapter 4 pertaining to diagnostic research. However, because one study rarely provides enough evidence to change clinical practice, you may need to review several studies. The Critical Appraisal Skills Programme (CASP) outlines 12 somewhat overlapping questions to aid in the appraisal of prognostic research. Using this tool will help you systematically determine the validity of the study,

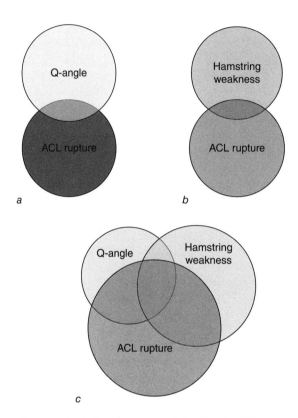

Figure 5.3 Venn diagram depicting factors contributing to ACL rupture.

the results, and whether the results will help you address your question.[4] Read the article, and then answer each question with *yes, no,* or *uncertain.* The questions are provided in the sidebar. After answering question 2, you will have completed an initial, or preliminary, review. If you answered *no* to the questions at this point, it may not be worth continuing to appraise the remainder of the article. Similar to the QUADAS assessment, there is no required number of *yes* answers; however, the greater the number of *yes* responses or explanations of *no* responses, the more trustworthy the study is.

Let's practice by reviewing the following article: Devan MR, Pescatello LS, Faghrit P, Anderson, A. A prospective study of overuse knee injuries among female athletes with muscle imbalance and structural abnormalities. *JAT.* 2004; 39 (3): 263-267.

In this scenario, you are a first-year athletic trainer at a new college. Your primary responsibility for sport coverage is women's soccer. The coach approaches you upon your arrival to the school and tells you that she is curious about the number of ACL and overuse injuries she has witnessed. She would like you to help develop a method to decrease the incidence. After performing a literature review using the Cochrane, PubMed, Medline, and CINAHL databases with the search terms *prognostic, prospective, ACL, overuse, injury, knees,* and *soccer,* you are going to read "A Prospective Study of Overuse Knee Injuries Among Female Athletes With Muscle Imbalance and Structural Abnormalities."[5] See the sidebar Critical Appraisal of Evidence on page 69 for more on this study.

Critical Appraisal Skills Programme (CASP) Questions

Answer each question as *yes*, *no*, or *uncertain*.

_____ 1. **Did the study address a clearly focused issue?** Did the authors clearly define the population and risk factors? Did the study try to detect a benefit or effect, and was this reported?

_____ 2. **Did the authors use an appropriate method to answer their question?** A prognostic study should use a cohort or case report. Are these appropriate methods for the question being reviewed?

_____ 3. **Was the cohort recruited in an acceptable way?** Was the selection of participants explained? Do they represent a defined population, and is that population representative of the population you are working with? Was there anything special about the population? Were all applicable persons included in the study?

_____ 4. **Was the exposure accurately measured to minimize bias?** Were subjective or objective measures used? Objective are preferred to minimize potential bias. Have the measures been validated?

_____ 5. **Was the outcome accurately measured to minimize bias?** Were outcomes measured subjectively or objectively? Has a reliable system been established for detecting the conditions of interest (disease, injury)? Were subjects and assessors blinded to the exposure or outcomes, and in this case, is that important?

_____ 6. **(a) Have the authors identified all important confounding factors? (b) Have they taken account of the confounding factors in the design or analysis?** Are there other confounding factors you can list? Has the author accounted for confounding factors in the design or results?

_____ 7. **(a) Was the follow-up of subjects complete enough? (b) Was the follow-up long enough?** Was follow-up thorough, and was it long enough to allow symptoms to present or resolve? Did the author report the number of people lost to follow up on? They may have had a different outcome.

(continued)

Critical Appraisal Skills Programme (CASP) Questions *(continued)*

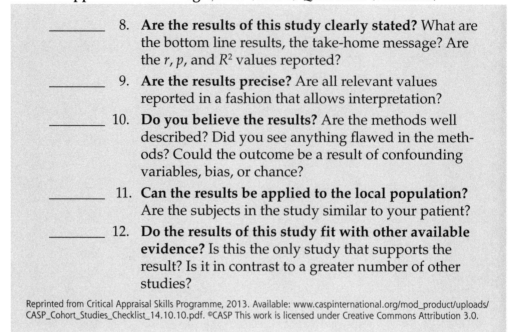

_____ 8. **Are the results of this study clearly stated?** What are the bottom line results, the take-home message? Are the r, p, and R^2 values reported?

_____ 9. **Are the results precise?** Are all relevant values reported in a fashion that allows interpretation?

_____ 10. **Do you believe the results?** Are the methods well described? Did you see anything flawed in the methods? Could the outcome be a result of confounding variables, bias, or chance?

_____ 11. **Can the results be applied to the local population?** Are the subjects in the study similar to your patient?

_____ 12. **Do the results of this study fit with other available evidence?** Is this the only study that supports the result? Is it in contrast to a greater number of other studies?

Reprinted from Critical Appraisal Skills Programme, 2013. Available: www.caspinternational.org/mod_product/uploads/CASP_Cohort_Studies_Checklist_14.10.10.pdf. ©CASP This work is licensed under Creative Commons Attribution 3.0.

After briefly reading the article for appropriateness, you decide to use the CASP to complete a thorough appraisal. Compare your answers to these sample answers:

- Item 1, Yes. The study clearly focused on the risk factors associated with female soccer athletes to include soccer and risk factors that might contribute to overuse injury.

- Item 2, Yes. This prospective study used a cohort of female NCAA athletes and took baseline measures at the start of the season that allowed the researchers to address the question of causes of overuse issues at the end of the season.

- Item 3, Yes. The cohort was representative of college female athletes and relates to the current topic at your new school. The author noted the conditions that excluded particular athletes who would otherwise have been included.

- Item 4, Yes. The Biodex provides an objective measure of strength. The goniometer and Ober's test are not perfect assessments, but the author details the procedures in reproducible detail.

- Item 5, Uncertain. The author states that the principal investigator collected the data on the Biodex, but refers to a primary investigator who measured Q angles and performed Ober's tests. It is unclear whether this is the same person. The author also states that the Q-angle measures and Ober's tests were performed once, and a single test might be less reliable than repeated tests.

- Item 6, Yes. The author clearly explains that injuries to the knee that occurred as a result of trauma were not classified as overuse, and clinical diagnosis was used throughout the season to track knee injuries.

- Item 7, Yes. The follow-up of subjects was thorough. The actual length of time into the season or length of the season itself was not recorded, but clinical

Critical Appraisal of Evidence

In this critical appraisal of evidence, we are evaluating the efficacy of this study to help you address the coach's concern. Let's begin with a brief review of the article.

Study Overview

The purpose of this study is to prospectively examine the influence of hamstring-to-quadriceps (H:Q) ratio and structural abnormalities on the prevalence of overuse knee injuries among female collegiate athletes.

Methods

A total of 53 healthy college females completed isokinetic H:Q strength ratio assessments at 60°/s and 300°/s on a Biodex system. Genu recurvatum and Q-angle measurements were assessed using a goniometer, and iliotibial flexibility was assessed using Ober's test. The reported results show an association between H:Q strength ratios and overuse injuries.

Critical Appraisal

1. Outcomes: During the course of the study, 10 overuse conditions occurred. Poor H:Q ratios were associated with more overuse knee injuries.

2. Deduction: It appears that strength and conditioning may be associated with overuse injuries. This is relevant to your situation. You decide to review the article further.

experience would suffice to say that a full season provides ample time to develop overuse injuries.

- Item 8, Yes. The bottom-line results are clear. The logical conclusion presented by the author is that female athletes who lack sufficient hamstring endurance relative to quadriceps endurance at 300°/sec exhibit predisposing factors to overuse knee injuries during the competitive season.

- Item 9, Yes. In this method of statistical review, confidence intervals are not recorded. The *p* values of hamstring-to-quadriceps endurance ratios at 300°/sec are significant and reported.

- Item 10, Yes. Confounding variables were accounted for, the primary outcome was based on objective data captured by the Biodex, and I would trust the recommendation to address hamstring endurance to potentially minimize overuse knee injuries.

- Items 11 and 12, Yes. The results of this study can be applied to help decrease the number of injuries on the soccer team. Evidence also suggests the importance of maintaining balance between the strength and endurance of the hamstrings and quadriceps.

Foundations of Evidence: Identifying Types of Studies

Here is a simple graphic to help you identify the type of study based on the aim, how the intervention was performed, and when the outcomes were determined.

Spotting the Study Design

The type of study can generally be identified by looking at three issues:

Q1. What was the aim of the study?

1. To simply describe a population (PO questions) → descriptive
2. To quantify the relationship between factors (PICO questions) → analytical

Q2. If analytical, was the intervention randomly allocated?

1. Yes → RCT
2. No → observational study

For observational studies, the main types will then depend on the timing of the measurement of outcome, so our third question is

Q3. When were the outcomes determined?

1. Some time after the exposure or intervention → cohort study (prospective study)
2. At the same time as the exposure intervention → cross-sectional study or survey
3. Before the exposure was determined → case control study (retrospective study based on recall of the exposure)

Reprinted from Center for Evidenced-Based Medicine, 2014. Available: www.cebm.net/study-designs/. This work is licensed under the Creative Commons – Attribution 4.0 International.

Summary

Prognostic simply means predicting or attempting to estimate the risk of future conditions. Prognostic research can be as intuitive as trying to minimize the risk of heatstroke when numerous variables would indicate such a risk. It allows you to take preventive measures and avoid potentially serious injuries or illnesses. Protecting athletes is at the very heart of what athletic trainers do. Athletics is also a perfect venue in which to perform cohort studies, because teams are natural cohorts, and athletes of the same sport across many institutions share very similar characteristics. Remember, predictions based on prognostic research are not intended to replace athletic trainers and allow coaches to perform our duties. Predictions based on prognostic research provide objective data to expand your clinical information and improve the care you provide to athletes.

References

1. Karel G, Moons M, Royston P, Vergouwe Y, Grobbee DE, Altman DG. Prognosis and prognostic research: What, why, and how? *BMJ*. 2009; 338. doi: 10.1136/bmj.b375.

2. Fetters LK, Tilson J. *Evidence based physical therapy.* Philadelphia: Davis; 2012.

3. Centre for Evidence-Based Medicine (CEBM). Making a decision. www.cebm.net/index.aspx?o=1854. Accessed June 1, 2014.

4. Critical Appraisal Skills Programme (CASP). Making sense of evidence. www.caspinternational.org/mod_product/uploads/CASP_Cohort_Studies_Checklist_14.10.10.pdf. Accessed June 2, 2014.

5. Devan M, Pescatello L, Faghri P, Anderson J. A prospective study of overuse knee injuries among female athletes with muscle imbalance and structural abnormalities. *JAT.* 2004; 39 (3): 263-267.

CHAPTER 6

Systematic Reviews and Meta-Analyses

Objectives

After reading this chapter, you will be able to do the following:

- Understand the advantages of finding evidence at the top of the evidence pyramid.
- Communicate the purposes of critically appraised topics, systematic reviews, and meta-analyses and how they differ.
- Understand how each type of research study is generally designed and conducted to be able to critically evaluate study outcomes.
- Perform an EBP search using systematic review and meta-analysis databases to answer your PICO question.

Now that you have an understanding of diagnostic and prognostic research approaches, it is time to look at how the preponderance of research studies within those areas can be combined to inform your evidence-based practice. The top three levels of the evidence pyramid are critically appraised individual articles, critically appraised topics, and systematic reviews that may include meta-analyses. These types of studies evaluate the outcomes of many individual studies on a particular topic to identify the outcomes with the highest quality of evidence supporting them. This chapter focuses on critically appraised topics, systematic reviews, and meta-analyses so that you understand the purposes of each, how they are conducted, and the resources available for finding each type of review. At the end of the chapter, you will choose a topic and perform an EBP search of systematic review databases to inform a clinical curiosity you may have.

Review of the Evidence Pyramid

The evidence pyramid was provided in chapter 1 (see figure 1.1). To understand the importance of **critically appraised topics (CATs)**, systematic reviews (SRs), and meta-analyses (MAs), we will now look at the pyramid in more detail. At the bottom of the pyramid are expert opinion articles. Although these are helpful for gaining a general understanding of a topic, they commonly do not provide any new evidence.

Above expert opinion are three levels of **unfiltered information**: case series reports, cohort studies, and randomized controlled trials (RCTs). *Unfiltered* simply means that the methods are not evaluated piece by piece in combination with other studies. RCTs are excellent resources for informing your clinical practice, because they represent individual research studies investigating particular topics. For example, if you were interested in methods to prevent medial tibial stress syndrome (MTSS), commonly referred to as shin splints, you could go to the PubMed database, type in your search terms, and find these RCTs. Some studies investigate one prevention method, whereas others investigate multiple methods. It is up to you to determine the quality of each study to decide whether to implement the prevention method in your practice. To that end, you would need to perform a critical appraisal of each study. If one of the studies looks at arch supports only in comparison with a control group (no treatment) and has only five subjects in each group, it would not be wise to consider implementing the method. If that same study had 45 subjects in each group, this would provide more valid and generalizable results to inform your practice. Of the study types at the unfiltered level of the evidence pyramid, RCTs provide the highest quality of evidence.

In the upper echelon of the evidence pyramid are three levels of **filtered information**: critically appraised individual articles, critically appraised topics (CATs), and systematic reviews (SRs), which typically include meta-analyses (MAs). Filtered information has been evaluated along with multiple similar studies by someone other than the researcher and then combined with those studies to form a comprehensive review of outcomes for a particular topic. In the evidence pyramid, CATs are typically below SRs, which include MAs. Although some sources put SRs and MAs at the same level, some differentiate between them and set meta-analyses at the very top of the evidence pyramid. Most often, systematic reviews include meta-analyses within the report. It is important to keep in mind that CATs, SRs, and MAs are not meant to replace basic research and observational studies, such as RCTs. Rather, their purpose is to condense the enormous number of related study outcomes on a topic, when appropriate.

Using our previous MTSS prevention example, numerous studies over the years have investigated whether stretching, arch support, strengthening, body mass index changes, and other things have any bearing on the occurrence of MTSS. A filtered review would condense all of the well-designed studies into an outcome measure to inform your clinical practice.

Definitions of and Differences Among Filtered Reviews

Filtered reviews allow clinicians to let statistical experts evaluate research articles around specific areas of interest and provide a summary of results. Our hope is that you will become proficient at finding and interpreting these relevant reviews. But to do that, you must have a clear understanding of what each of the three filtered review types offers.

Critically Appraised Individual Article and Topics

Critically appraised individual articles provide a thorough assessment of one study. They answer questions such as Were the methods solid? Were the results and conclusions appropriate? Are the results generalizable? and Do the results suggest that further research is needed? These synopses are helpful when there is not a lot of research for a particular topic that can be combined in a CAT.

CATs came about with the advent of online accessibility of research articles. Critically appraised topics are "a one-page summary of the literature appraisal and clinical relevance of a specific clinical topic."[1] CATs are a bit unique in that any clinician or researcher can enter certain study aspects into a program to create a CAT. To date, CATmaker is the prominent electronic program serving this purpose. The helpful thing about CATs is that they are truly one-page summaries of relevant articles on a topic of interest. That said, there may not be a CAT for every athletic training clinical condition you may be curious about. Further, because many clinicians create their own CATs and share them perhaps only with their peers or work groups, many CATs do not make it into electronic databases where other clinicians around the world can find them.

Similar to CATs are best evidence topics (BETs). These typically include a few articles on a topic, but fewer than six as a general rule.[2] BETs and CATs are used interchangeably at times. The Centre for Evidence-Based Medicine (CEBM) links directly to a BET database (BestBET). CAT databases, meanwhile, are harder to find because CATs are commonly made and stored by individual clinicians.

Systematic Reviews

Systematic reviews (SRs) have been around for decades, although the statistical analysis function has matured a great deal. Systematic reviews are "scientific tools that can be used to appraise, summarize, and communicate the results and implications of otherwise unmanageable quantities of research."[3] For example, if you performed an EBP search in PubMed or CINAHL for *ankle instability and rehabilitation,* you would find thousands of research articles. No one has time to read thousands of research articles, much less critically appraise each one. Thus, the need for systematic reviews arose. SRs attempt to be objective in their interpretation of studies and have reproducible conclusions. Whereas CATs review only a few research articles per topic, SRs strive to include almost every research article that is relevant to the topic at hand. This means all of those thousands of articles on ankle instability and rehabilitation! At times, SRs include meta-analyses if the research study methods and outcome measures are similar enough from study to study that combining the outcomes makes clinical sense.

Meta-Analyses

Meta-analyses (MAs) are statistical combinations of several research study outcomes or results to produce an estimate of the effect of an intervention. **Effect size** is a value that reflects the magnitude of the treatment effect or the strength of the relationship between two variables.[4] However, to synthesize the statistics of many research studies, each study must have an effect size statistic computed. To complicate matters, effect sizes may be reported or computed using different statistical methods. A discussion of different effect size measures, however, is beyond the scope of this text. The complexity in combining different effect size measures tends to limit the number of MAs conducted.

Meta-analyses "are a specific statistical strategy for assembling the results of several studies into a single estimate."[3] The difficulty in combining study outcomes is that studies use different outcome measures to assess the efficacy of a treatment. For example, when deciding whether to advise a baseball athlete to have rotator cuff surgery or to avoid surgery and go through conservative treatment, you can use various outcome measures to determine which route is better. One study may look at how long pain lasted through rehabilitation in each intervention. Another may look at the outcome of time to return to play. Another may look at the reinjury rate. Yet another may look at pitching accuracy and speed (performance) compared to preinjury measures. Combining these studies into one MA would not work. Conversely, studies that compared various rotator cuff surgical techniques using the same outcome measure of reinjury rates could and should be compared through an MA. Each of those studies would need to have its statistical outcome measure computed into an effect size. Then the effect size statistics would be combined to form one summary effect statistic.[4]

Strengths and Processes of Critically Appraised Topics (CATs)

The strengths of CATs are that they are easy to read and any clinician or researcher can input data into a program such as CATmaker to create a CAT. Clinicians can then build their own CAT libraries. This makes CATs very popular. They are typically one-page summaries of some of the most pertinent research studies on a topic. However, keep in mind that CATs do not summarize all of the research on any topic as systematic reviews do. This limits their usefulness at times. With CATs, you must be aware of statistical measures that demonstrate the validity and significance of the reported outcomes. Figure 6.1 shows an output from a search for CATs on chronic ankle instability.

Design Methods and Outcome Measures

CATs are created by beginning with a clinically relevant question in PICO format. You perform a regular EBP search using this question (if you are intending to create a CAT), or use a CAT search engine (if you are hoping to find a published CAT about your topic). To create a CAT, once you have a few pertinent research articles that answer your question, you input information into a CAT creation program such as CATmaker. The program will ask for your PICO elements, your search strategy, and key statistical elements from each relevant study you found. From there, the program automatically calculates clinically useful measures that affect the final outcome. This summary helps you to formulate clinical practice guidelines from each of the articles you included in the CAT. The program also automatically creates a CAT file that you can share with colleagues. Each CAT has six components that clarify the clinical question and its relevance, summarize and appraise the evidence, and end with application to athletes and citations—all within one page.

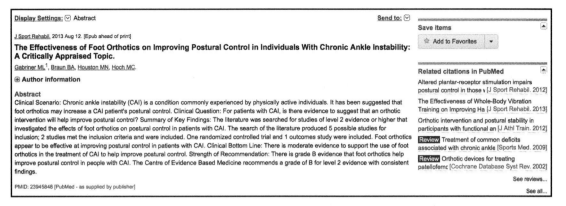

Figure 6.1   CAT article on chronic ankle instability.
Reprinted from PubMed.gov. Available: www.ncbi.nlm.nih.gov/pubmed.

Foundations of Evidence: Components of a Critically Appraised Topic (CAT)

1. Clinical question
2. Clinical bottom line (clinical implications for the athlete)
3. Summary of key evidence
4. Appraisal of the evidence study or studies
5. Applicability to the athlete
6. Citations

When Are CATs Appropriate to Use?

CATs are appropriate to use when you need quick answers to common questions. For example, if you wanted to know whether thermal ultrasound is the best treatment option for subacute patellar tendinitis, you could quickly enter that search into a CAT search engine or metasearch engine to find an answer. Numerous CATs are available to aid the clinical practice of athletic trainers. Thus, you are encouraged to get into one of the CAT search engines and practice searching for CATs. Remember, not every athletic training clinical situation or condition will have an associated CAT. Some of the less common injuries and treatments that we work with in the athletic training room fall into this category. Additionally, because any clinician with a CAT creation program can create a CAT on any topic, you should only use CATs from sources you trust.

If you work in a setting that attracts a particular type of athlete consistently, then you may want to acquire CATmaker so you can create and share your own library of CATs. For example, if you work at a high school or middle school, you may want to investigate treatment options for injuries that are specific to youth athletes. If you work in a collegiate setting, you may want to create CATs specific to the presurgical treatment of various injuries. If you work in a hospital outpatient clinic, it may be wise to create CATs for the geriatric population, perhaps specific to joint replacement rehabilitation guidelines.

When Are CATs Not Appropriate to Use?

CATs are not helpful when dealing with complex or previously unanswered questions. For example, a CAT would not be appropriate for seeking the best treatment methods for athletes with medial tibial stress syndrome (MTSS), because there are no proven EBP treatment methods to date. Searching in a CAT database for this question would yield no hits. Thus, you would need to do a full EBP search and evaluate the quality of the research articles on your own using critical appraisal tools. From that, you determine which treatments for MTSS may show some promise, even if the study results are not reproducible.

Strengths and Processes of Systematic Reviews (SRs)

Systematic reviews (SRs) are particularly helpful because they condense large numbers of research articles and synthesize their results. Often, the results of the individual articles may contradict each other, which is typically reflected in the SR conclusions. SRs are large undertakings that require trained researchers to conduct them. Therein lies their merit—each SR is a cumulative recommendation from as close to 100% of the research on that topic as the research team can ensure. Thus, when you read an SR, you can fairly accurately assume that almost all of the available relevant evidence on that topic was considered. However, you still need to evaluate the methods used to conduct the SR via a systematic review appraisal, which is presented in more detail in a later section.

Design Methods and Outcome Measures

Systematic reviews are conducted through a very rigorous methodology. The Cochrane Collaboration initially developed this process, which is followed by most

Foundations of Evidence: Steps of a Systematic Review

1. Define an appropriate question.
2. Search the literature.
3. Define the inclusion and exclusion criteria, and select articles for inclusion in the review.
4. Evaluate and report the quality of each included study.
5. Combine the results into an aggregated summary.
6. Place the findings in context.

researchers today.[5] The sidebar Foundations of Evidence: Steps of a Systematic Review lists the six general steps in the SR development process.[3,6]

The first step is to define an appropriate question. A good question to ask is Why is this clinical question important to answer? The question should very clearly define the population or athletes, the intervention, and appropriate outcomes. A high-quality SR has each of these components clearly stated. If the population or athletes have an injury that has varying degrees of progression, that must be defined in this initial step. For example, if researching the surgical treatment of SLAP lesions (superior labrum anterior to posterior), it would be important to define which grade of lesions will be included in the study. A grade 1 lesion may not involve enough damage to the labrum to warrant surgery at all.

The second step is to perform a full, exhaustive search. This should include studies that are both published and unpublished, RCTs, studies in all languages, and so on. Reference lists of all major articles should be reviewed to find other articles that may inform the SR. At the end of this second step, you should be confident that all relevant studies have been considered.

The third step in the SR development process is to create study inclusion and exclusion criteria and choose the studies to include. A systematic and standardized approach should be used to appraise the studies to avoid biases. To that end, at least two reviewers should work independently to review each article for inclusion or exclusion, based on the criteria. Following their independent reviews, the reviewers should come together to finalize the list of studies to be included in the SR. You will see as you read more SRs that the initial study number is usually well into the hundreds or thousands. But by the time the independent researchers combine their inclusion and exclusion results, the number of studies drops dramatically.

Step 4 requires experienced researchers to evaluate the quality of each included study. The quality or validity (or both) of each study should be commented on in the SR, either within the text or, more commonly, in a table. An assessment of the risk of biases is included in this step to gauge the quality of the evidence in a more refined way. Biases either exaggerate or underestimate the true effect of an intervention.[6] Figure 6.2 shows a summary assessment of studies in table format within an SR.

The fifth step, combining the results, may include a meta-analysis if appropriate. The results of the included articles are combined to create a summary estimate of the overall effect of the interventions in question. Some SRs present this in a qualitative manner, but more commonly it is presented in the form of a quantitative MA. The MA process is defined in the following MA section. MAs should be performed only when the studies are similar in terms of athletes or populations, interventions, and outcomes. MA outcomes are usually provided in the form of a forest plot and a summary measure of effect size with a confidence interval (figure 6.3).

The final step in an SR requires placing the findings in context. This includes a discussion of the quality and heterogeneity of the included studies, the likely impact of

Table 3 Summary of intervention effects			
Interventions/outcome	Time to recovery	Global perceived effect	Pain
Iontophoresis, phonophoresis, ultrasound therapy or ice massage versus control	NA	NA	+
Iontophoresis versus phonophoresis, ice massage and ultrasound therapy	NA	NA	+/−
Periosteal pecking versus ultrasound therapy	NA	NA	+ or +/−
Low-energy laser versus sham laser	NA	+/−	+/−
Brace versus no brace	+/−	+/−	+/−
Pulsed electromagnetic field versus placebo	NA	+/−	+/−
ESWT versus control treatment	+	+	+

+ Indicates a positive effect, − indicates a negative effect, +/− indicates no effect, *ESWT* extracorporeal shockwave therapy, *NA* not applicable

Figure 6.2 Summary assessment of included studies in a systematic review.

Reprinted from Springer.com. Available: http://link.springer.com.

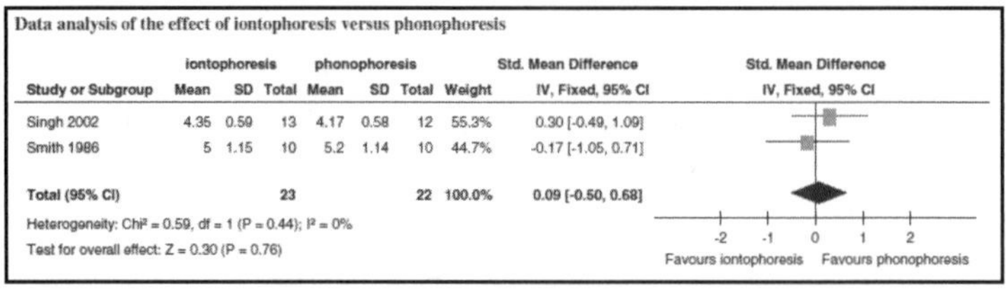

Figure 6.3   Forest plot of iontophoresis versus phonophoresis.
Reprinted from Springer.com. Available: http://link.springer.com.

any biases, and the applicability of the findings to the intended athletes. This section of the SR is possibly the most important to read and understand, because it will imply how useful the outcomes of the SR are to your evidence-based practice. Do not be surprised if some of the SRs that you encounter report that there is not enough high-quality evidence to come to any conclusion about the topic. At times, this is because a majority of the included studies were methodologically flawed; at other times it is simply because each of the included studies showed no significant findings.

When Are SRs Appropriate to Use?

Incorporating research evidence into practice can be time-consuming. Systematic reviews facilitate this process by rigorously synthesizing the results of numerous studies into a useful summary. These reviews are appropriate to use whenever you come across a condition that has had great attention in research journals, but with conflicting results. Because they are at the top of the evidence pyramid, commonly including meta-analyses, SRs should be a common pursuit. When you have created a PICO question and are ready to enter it into database queries, search engines, or both, it would be wise to include some of the SR search engines listed in the section How to Find Critically Appraised Topics, Systematic Reviews, and Meta-Analyses later in this chapter. You may discover that many of the research studies you find are already included in one SR.

If you are considering using an SR in your practice, you need to be sure that it was conducted with integrity and thoroughness. A quick critical appraisal can be done by asking four general questions.[5,7] The first is as follows: *Did the review explicitly address a specific and clear question?* The second question is this: *Did your search results include studies that were detailed, thorough, and exhaustive?* The search methodology should be explicitly addressed within the SR. The third critical appraisal question is the following: *Were the included studies of high methodological quality?* Last and most important, you should ask whether the selection and assessments of the included studies were reproducible. If another group of researchers were to take on the same clinical question to perform an SR, would they come up with the same studies and results? If the answer to this last question is no, then the SR you are assessing may be of low quality.

When Are SRs Not Appropriate to Use?

Systematic reviews are appropriate to use for any treatment intervention. If no SR exists for your PICO question, then you will need to rely on all of the individual studies that result from your search. Unfortunately, not every treatment intervention

Foundations of Evidence:
Steps for a Critical Appraisal of a Systematic Review

1. Is the clinical question focused?
2. Was the literature search thorough and exhaustive?
3. Are the included studies of high quality and valid?
4. Is the selection of the included studies reproducible?

has been addressed by an SR (e.g., conditions that have a clear, noncontroversial, proven treatment). For people with plantar fasciitis, the most common treatment intervention is orthotics. This is so widely accepted and proven to be effective in research studies that performing an SR would likely do nothing more than confirm the already accepted treatment. Generally speaking, whenever a high-quality SR is available, it is appropriate to use.

Strengths and Processes of Meta-Analyses (MAs)

Meta-analyses are at the very top of the evidence pyramid, within systematic reviews. However, because they have a very specific function, they should be performed only within the framework of carefully conducted systematic reviews. Their function is to produce precise statistical estimates of the effect of an intervention on a certain condition.[8] In other words, MAs are meant to make your clinical practice more efficient and effective. That said, MAs have come under scrutiny, because they do not necessarily control for biases in the included research studies or for how the results were disseminated (publication bias).[9] In fact, the PRISMA Statement (Preferred Reporting Items for Systematic Reviews and Meta-Analyses) clearly states that "the failure of a systematic review [and/or meta-analysis] to report the assessment of the risk of bias in included studies may be seen as a marker of poor conduct, given the importance of this activity in the systematic review process."[7] So, when an MA is used within an SR, always make sure that the authors evaluated the risk of various biases. These evaluations are typically presented in a graph or table format.

Design Methods and Outcome Measures

MAs should be performed only when the included studies in an SR are similar in terms of population or athletes, interventions, and outcomes. There are generally two steps in the creation of an MA.[3] The first step is to extract outcome data from each included study. An effect size is then calculated for each study from that data. With that effect size statistic, a **confidence interval** (an estimate of the chance variation expected with similar studies) is also calculated.

The second step in performing an MA is determining whether it is appropriate to calculate a pooled average, or summary effect, of the effect sizes across the included studies. If so, then that pooled average should be presented. Care needs to be taken here to be certain that the studies are indeed similar enough in athletes, intervention, and outcome measures to validate the pooled summary effect statistic as the estimate of the overall effect of the intervention.

For example, if an SR were designed to evaluate all studies pertaining to the effect the type of playing surface had on knee injury rate, the MA could be performed only if the same outcome measure of a specific knee injury was used—such as meniscal injury. Because there are many types of knee injuries that may have nothing to do with playing surface, all of the surfaces could not be combined with all of the knee injuries to produce an MA. Having one clearly defined outcome measure is important to qualify an MA.

As mentioned earlier, MA outcomes are usually provided in the form of a forest plot and a reported effect size with a confidence interval (see figure 6.3). In a forest plot, the vertical line is the line of no effect. Each study plotted to the right of the vertical line usually favors the intervention in question. Each study plotted to the left of the line usually favors the control group or the nonsignificance of the intervention in question. If the study is comparing two interventions, the vertical line is the line of equal effect, with one side of the line favoring one intervention and other side of the line favoring the other intervention. The short, thin horizontal lines that represent each study indicate the length of the confidence intervals. The longer the line (and confidence interval) is, the less precise the study results are.[10] Finally, the larger symbol at the bottom of the vertical line indicates the pooled summary effect statistic. Thus, forest plots provide a quick visual representation of how many included studies favored the intervention (and by how much) and how many showed no significant difference between the intervention group and the control group—or perhaps favored an opposing treatment rather than a control group. In figure 6.3, the opposing intervention is depicted on the right side.

When Are MAs Appropriate to Use?

MAs are appropriate to use when combining the statistics in several studies that have similar athletes, interventions, and outcomes. They are also appropriate when conducted within a well-designed systematic review. Because MAs are data reduction tools, they are not stand-alone pieces of work. They fit within the grander systematic review framework. Thus, you would not be able to search specifically for an MA on a particular topic. Rather, you would search for an SR on that topic and see whether an MA was conducted within that review. Nevertheless, MAs are considered to be the highest-quality marker of evidence, per the evidence pyramid.

When Are MAs Not Appropriate to Use?

MAs are not useful when the included studies are fraught with biases. A high-quality SR that includes an MA will address the potential biases within the review. If this is not apparent when reading an SR with an MA, use great caution when interpreting the results of the MA. Additionally, if you find that an MA compares studies that do not have similar athletes or populations, interventions, and outcomes, then the MA is not valid. For example, if you were researching the previous chronic ankle instability example and found many articles on medial ligament insufficiency and several others on only lateral ligament insufficiency, combining all of those article outcomes into one MA would be inappropriate, because the injuries are different. So be certain when reviewing an SR with an included MA that the studies are similar in terms of athletes, interventions, and especially outcome measures.

How to Find Critically Appraised Topics, Systematic Reviews, and Meta-Analyses

With a basic understanding of the definitions, purposes, and processes used to create CATs, SRs, and MAs, you are ready to dive into the literature to find some of these reports to inform your EBP. The most helpful resources are databases and search engines that are specific to these types of reports. CAT Crawler is the most helpful CAT-finding tool; the Cochrane Library houses the most extensive and well-reviewed systematic reviews and their meta-analyses.

Finding CATs

CAT Crawler (developed by Singapore's Bioinformatics Institute) is defined as a metasearch engine. It has been evaluated quantitatively and found to be more thorough and precise than individual CAT search engines. Individual CAT search engines include BestBET (developed by the Emergency Department, Manchester Royal Infirmary) and Evidence-Based Pediatrics (developed by the Department of Pediatrics, University of Michigan Health System, Ann Arbor).[11]

Finding Systematic Reviews and Meta-Analyses

The Cochrane Library, or the Cochrane Collaboration, is the most comprehensive collection of regularly updated SRs in the allied health and medical professions.[10] This library is the gold standard search engine for the best quantity and quality of SRs. The Collaboration prepares, maintains, and promotes SRs to inform health care decisions.[5] Further, it is easily accessible through any university library research web page or by simply entering *Cochran Collaboration* into the search bar of your web browser.

PubMed Health also specializes in systematic reviews of clinical effectiveness research.[12] This site includes SR abstracts from both DARE (Database of Abstracts of Reviews of Effects) and the Cochrane Collaboration. DARE itself contains some SRs and many RCTs.

One of the most powerful metasearch engines is TRIP (Translating Research Into Practice). TRIP searches several databases simultaneously to find every type of evidence from randomized controlled trials to systematic reviews. As of this writing, TRIP searches over 25 medical and EBP databases.[13] TRIP is easy to access and easy to use.

Practice EBP Searches

Finding evidence for a clinical question you have should be getting a bit easier for you at this point. What will improve your clinical practice further is to be able to find critically appraised topics (or best evidence topics), systematic reviews, and meta-analyses—all at the very top of the evidence pyramid. By using the evidence from these sources, you can be much more confident that what you have is a more thorough synthesis of the evidence rather than individual RCTs that you need to critically appraise on your own. So, it's time to practice!

Create a PICO question that you may have seen outcomes for previously in individual research studies. If you are struggling to create a question, consider the following:

- **Scenario 1.** Does stretching the lower leg or supporting the arch work better to treat medial tibial stress syndrome in runners? With this scenario, because there may be little to no treatment methods that are proven to work for MTSS beyond rest, you may want to start with fewer search terms, such as *medial tibial stress syndrome AND treatment.* If you get too many results from this, then simply add more specific search terms.
- **Scenario 2.** Do basketball players with patellar tendinosis return to play more quickly with conservative treatment or with surgical treatment? You could change the outcome measure from *time to return to play* to *reinjury rates* if that's more in line with your athlete's goals and values.
- **Scenario 3.** Do American football players with diagnosed concussions that include vestibulocochlear deficits have a quicker resolution of concussion symptoms with complete rest or with vestibulocochlear rehabilitation combined with rest? Because the vestibulocochlear rehabilitation of concussed athletes is fairly new, you may need to be less specific, using the terms *concussion AND treatment* first and then narrowing that down to include *vestibulocochlear* as appropriate.

Figure 6.4 shows the search results from entering the search terms for scenario 1 into the Cochrane Collaboration search bar. Remember that not everything we do in the athletic training room has evidence to support it—much less enough evidence to warrant performing an SR. However, thanks to the Cochrane Collaboration, the number of SRs is increasing.

With your PICO question in hand, use Cochrane Collaboration, PubMed Health, and TRIP to determine which has more evidence on your topic and whether those studies are SRs and MAs or simply RCTs. For scenario 1, figures 6.4, 6.5, and 6.6 illustrate the results from each of these search engines.

Once you find an SR (hopefully) on your topic, you should critically appraise it using the following four questions:

1. Is the clinical question focused?
2. Was the literature search thorough and exhaustive?
3. Are the included studies of high quality and valid?
4. Is the selection of the included studies reproducible?

From your search, choose one of the systematic reviews and highlight where in the review each of these questions is addressed. You are simply looking for a yes or no answer to each of the four questions. If any of the questions has a no answer, then the quality of the SR is lower, and you should interpret its results with great caution. As you get more practice with this, you will become more proficient at determining the quality of the SR during your initial reading.

Once your critical appraisal is complete, it is time to determine if and how you intend to implement the outcomes of the SR into your clinical practice, perhaps

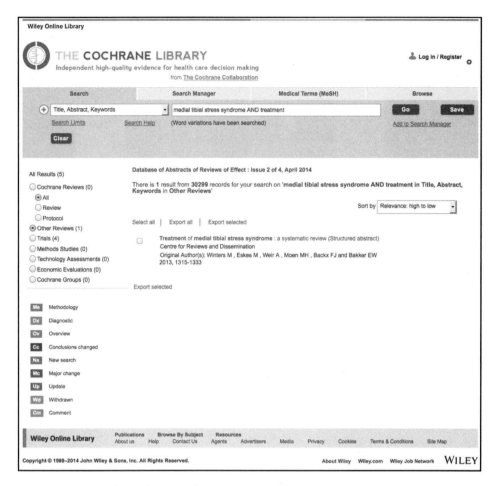

Figure 6.4 Search results in Cochrane Collaboration.
Reprinted from The Cochrane Library. Available: onlinelibrary.wiley.com/cochranelibrary/search.

with an athlete you are working with. Recall that implementing evidence into clinical practice is a combination of finding the evidence, weighing your own clinical experience with the topic, and weighing your athlete's values and needs.

For example, with the MTSS example, the treatment that has shown the greatest promise is extracorporeal shockwave therapy (ECSWT). This tool is not available in many athletic training rooms. Thus, you would need to refer your athlete to a physician who uses ECSWT. Additionally, the treatments are successive over several weeks, many insurance companies do not cover ECSWT, and it's expensive. Thus, although your EBP search may have yielded a great systematic review that did provide a treatment for MTSS that is evidence based, this treatment may not be desirable for your athlete. This would send you back to your SR of choice to see if there was a close second treatment for MTSS. Then you and your athlete would consider that option. Remember that at the end of your search, the SR may not have evidence to support any one direction. That in itself is informative, although certainly not ideal. As you become more efficient at finding SRs, your ability to

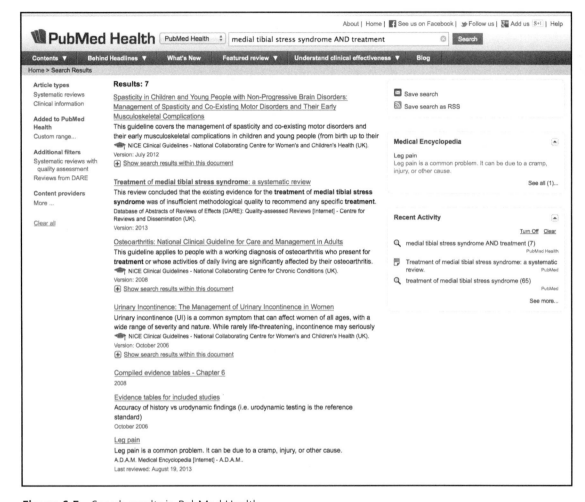

Figure 6.5 Search results in PubMed Health.
Reprinted from PubMed.gov. Available: www.ncbi.nlm.nih.gov/pubmed.

find quality reviews that change your clinical practice and produce more positive results will increase.

Summary

This chapter revisited the full evidence pyramid to provide a better understanding of the evidence at the very top of the pyramid—the filtered information types. These types of studies—critically appraised topics (and best evidence topics), systematic reviews, and meta-analyses—provide a mechanism for dealing with the preponderance of research studies available in the literature by condensing them to better inform your clinical practice. Each of the three types of filtered information was reviewed in detail to define its purposes, how it is conducted, and when it is appropriate and perhaps inappropriate to use. Toward the end of the chapter, resources in which to find each type of review were introduced. Finally, you were

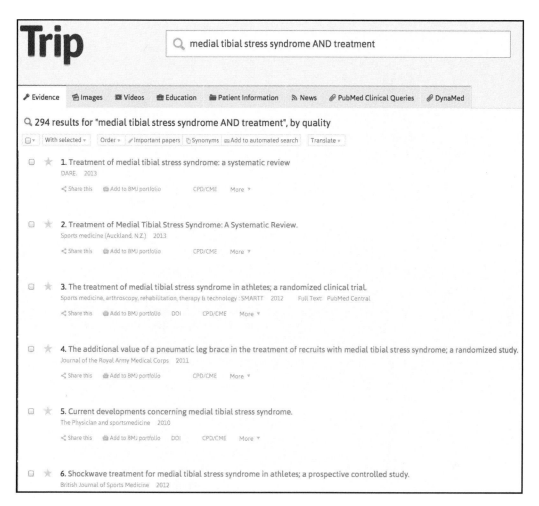

Figure 6.6 Search results in TRIP.

Reprinted from Turning Research Into Practice (TRIP) 2014.

asked to perform EBP searches within three of those databases so that you could practice finding and interpreting systematic reviews. We hope that you can now begin to use these reviews in your practice to improve athlete care.

References

1. Crowell M, Tragord B, Taylor A, Deyle G. Integration of critically appraised topics into evidence-based physical therapist practice. *J Orthop Sports Phys Ther*. 2012; 42 (10): 870-879.

2. Oxford Centre for Evidence-Based Medicine (CEBM) scale. www.cebm.net/index.aspx?o=1157. Updated 2013. Accessed March 30, 2014.

3. Green S. Systematic reviews and meta-analyses. *Singapore Med J*. 2005; 46 (6): 270-275.

4. Borenstein M, Hedges LV, Higgins JPT, Rothstein HR. *Introduction to meta-analysis.* West Sussex, UK: Wiley, 2011: 421.

5. Cochrane Library. www.cochranelibrary.com/view/0/index.html. Updated 2014. Accessed March 30, 2014.

6. Khan K, Kunz R, Kleijnen J, Antes G. Five steps to conducting a systematic review. *J R Soc Med.* 2003; 96: 118-122.

7. Moher D, Liberati A, Tetzlaff J, Altman D. Preferred reporting items for systematic reviews and meta-analyses: The PRISMA statement. *Ann Intern Med.* 2009; 151 (4): 264-265.

8. Egger M, Smith G, Sterne J, et al. Systematic reviews and meta-analysis. In: *Methods of public health.* Vol. 2. 5th ed. Oxford, UK: Oxford University Press, 2009: 623-641.

9. Egger M, Smith G, Schneider M, Minder C. Bias in meta-analysis detected by a simple graphical test. *BMJ.* 1997; 315: 629-639.

10. Reid K. Interpreting and understanding meta-analysis graphs: A practical guide. *Austr Fam Phys.* 2006; 35 (8): 635-644.

11. Dong P, Wong LL, Ng S, Loh M, Mondry A. Quantitative evaluation of recall and precision of CAT Crawler, a search engine specialized on retrieval of critically appraised topics. *BMC Med Inform Decis Mak.* 2004; 4: 21.

12. PubMed. www.ncbi.nlm.nih.gov/pubmed. Updated 2014. Accessed March 30, 2014.

13. Turning Research Into Practice (TRIP). www.tripdatabase.com. Updated 2014. Accessed March 30, 2014.

CHAPTER 7

EBP in Daily Clinical Practice

Objectives

After reading this chapter, you will be able to do the following:

- Assimilate your EBP research skills into your everyday clinical practice.
- Update your regular clinical practice techniques to include the latest evidence.
- Understand the importance of considering your athletes' values and needs when making daily clinical decisions.

With the wealth of information presented in the previous chapters, it's time to take a realistic look at how this can all fit into your daily clinical practice. Most practitioners have a fairly routine schedule. Adding another type of practice, such as performing EBP searches, will require a conscious effort. This chapter offers techniques to consider when tying all of the EBP information into various aspects of your daily practice. We will look at your practice based on evidence, your previous clinical experiences, and your athletes' values. Considering each of these components is critical to providing the best care possible. Change is hard to accept for many. However, evidence-based practice is here to stay, and we all must morph our practice into this new age.

Your Practice Based on Evidence

Consider this scenario: It's a busy afternoon in the athletic training room. As you're finishing up the treatment records for the soccer team, the football team begins to arrive for prepractice treatment and taping. One of your students asks you to evaluate a new injury on one of your quarterbacks. Before you're finished with that evaluation, another is waiting. Then the coach walks in asking for an update on his linemen. In typical triage fashion, you handle everything efficiently—including jotting down quick injury evaluation notes, setting up treatments, and updating coaches. Before you know it, you're almost late to practice. So you and your students load your equipment into the cart and head out to practice.

How many of us have gone through this scenario, and how often? It's almost common daily practice in the athletic training room in any setting. Within that routine, then, where are you supposed to take time out to do a quick EBP search on whether that subacute rotator cuff strain in your quarterback should be treated with pulsed or thermal ultrasound? Perhaps you questioned that when setting up his treatment but just relied on your clinical experience to make the decision. Does your clinical experience include EBP searches on this particular topic? If not, then it's time to make an EBP search a top priority.

Barriers to Implementing EBP Skills

When we ask clinicians what they believe the barriers are to implementing EBP into their daily practices, the most common response is lack of time.[1] Time is something we may all wish we had a little more of to complete those to-do lists. But in the athletic training setting, our schedules usually have some degree of flexibility. For example, in the preceding scenario regarding treating football players, updating coaches, and getting out to practice, the ideal time to perform that EBP search would be immediately after the evaluation and before applying the treatment. However, prepractice schedules rarely allow you time to step away and perform an EBP search. Fortunately, with the advent of smartphones and tablets, you may be able to perform that search once you get out to the field and practice is rolling. If you'd rather have eyes on the field, have one of your students perform the search as she's standing with you. She will certainly learn new information by performing the search too.

Another remedy to the time dilemma is to set time aside each morning when your athletic training room is closed to perform your EBP searches. Keep a list of topics or questions you're interested in on your desk, and attend to that list routinely. Also, remember that, as you practice searching, you will become more efficient and your searches will require less time. Other barriers to implementing EBP skills into your daily practice are presented in table 7.1, along with some possible solutions.[1,2]

Strategies to Enhance the Use of EBP

Having considered barriers to implementing EBP skills, along with some proposed solutions to those barriers, you can now consider strategies for gaining further knowledge of EBP. Some strategies identified in the literature specific to athletic training are seeking more EBP resources, gaining access to more preappraised resources (such as critically appraised topics and systematic reviews), attending EBP-specific workshops, engaging in peer discussions and mentorship regarding EBP, and gaining more experience simply by performing EBP searches until you are comfortable with the process.[3] Reading this text and taking the accompanying CEU quizzes are large steps toward enhancing your own evidence-based practice.

Putting Your EBP Search Results to Use

Once you have committed to making time daily to perform EBP searches that are directly applicable to the athletes you are working with, your next step is to assess whether your search results are usable with your athlete. Do the studies you found match your athlete's situation? To answer this question, you need to ask four basic questions.

Table 7.1 Common Barriers to Implementing EBP

Barriers	Solutions
Lack of time	Perform EBP searches in the mornings when AT rooms are slower or out at practices via mobile devices.
Lack of equipment and access to literature	With a computer and Internet access, most of the resources presented in this text are freely accessible at no cost.
Lack of generalizability of research	Look for larger studies; change search parameters to match your athlete's situation more closely.
Lack of research knowledge	Remember that you just need to be a consumer of research—not a researcher. Chapter 3 reviews research knowledge.
Lack of understanding of statistics	Chapter 9 reviews basic statistical measures that can help you interpret research findings.
Lack of search and appraisal skills	Chapter 2 addresses search basics; chapters 4 through 6 provide appraisal basics. Learning EBP search and appraisal skills takes practice, so give yourself time to get comfortable.
Lack of information resources	This text presents free resources.
EBP culture not well established in AT	You are at the forefront of helping to establish this culture!

The first question is whether the study participants were similar to your athlete. For example, if the randomized controlled trial (RCT) you found looked at baseball pitchers with rotator cuff tears, this would not be directly applicable to your quarterback with a rotator cuff tear, because they represent different populations whose throwing mechanics load the cuff differently. The baseball study may still inform your practice in other ways, however.

The second question to ask is whether your athlete matches the inclusion criteria of the study or studies you found. For example, if you found a systematic review of all overhead athletes with rotator cuff tears that considered whether ultrasound affected their time to return to play, your athlete would match the inclusion criteria. Be cautious when comparing study results of surgical populations to your athlete if your athlete is not having surgery to treat the condition—even if you are simply looking at a common treatment such as ultrasound. Comparing surgical patients to nonsurgical patients is a common mistake.

Foundations of Evidence: Determining Whether to Implement EBP Findings

1. Were the study participants similar to your athlete?
2. Does your athlete match the inclusion criteria?
3. Were all clinically important outcomes considered?
4. Are the likely benefits worth the risks of implementing the treatment?

Next, ask yourself if clinically important outcomes were considered in the study. This means asking if the outcome measures used in the study are relevant to your clinical question and your athlete. For example, a study looking at how exercise affects quality of life in a geriatric population is likely not clinically important to your population if you're working in the high school athletic training setting. In athletic training, our EBP searches will generally include clinically important outcomes, such as return to play, pain levels, and reinjury rates. A rotator cuff study that assesses return to activities of daily living versus return to playing sports may not be assessing an outcome that is clinically appropriate for your athlete.

Additionally, many studies include a measure of **minimal clinically important difference** (MCID) or **minimal detectable change** (MDC). Any MCID measure reported should include consideration of the gold standard used to define meaningful change in the population studied. A confidence interval should be reported so that you can determine whether the results of the MCID or the MDC measure are replicable with that level of confidence (commonly 95% confidence).

Finally, you should ask yourself whether the benefits of implementing the treatment outweigh the risks. There is rarely conflict with this question regarding typical athletic training practice, because we do not typically apply treatments that could cause harm. However, conversations with your athletes who may be considering whether to have surgery may require you to perform EBP searches to inform you and your athlete about the possible outcomes of each option. Other common risks that may outweigh the benefits deal with treatment timing when considering losing playing time, missing games, or perhaps missing the remainder of a season. For example, if an athlete with chronic plantar fasciitis is offered an injection by the team physician that would require five to seven days of no impact on the fascia, the athlete may choose to avoid the injection so that she can participate in the play-off game that weekend. The risk of not being recovered in time to play in the game may outweigh the benefit of playing without pain at a later date. The situations this last question addresses commonly involve the consideration of your athletes' values, which we discuss in more depth later in the chapter.

Dealing With Conflicting Evidence or No Evidence

It is not uncommon to find similar randomized controlled trials (RCTs) that have conflicting results—even within well-controlled studies. For example, if you were to perform an EBP search on risk factors for medial tibial stress syndrome (MTSS), you would find studies that report significant correlation with foot pronation (or navicular drop) and others that report no significant correlation with foot pronation (table 7.2). In fact, within this topic, one researcher has performed well-controlled studies and had opposite statistically significant results at different points in time.

So what do we do as clinicians when our search results in conflicting outcomes? If this happens, you need to rely on your critical appraisal of each article. If one article has 300 participants with matching relevant characteristics per group, and the conflicting article has 13 participants with matching relevant characteristics per group, you can consider the larger study to be more generalizable and have more power. If one of the studies mirrors your athlete's situation in terms of the PICO components more closely, then put more weight into considering the outcomes of

Table 7.2 Conflicting Results From EBP Search

Studies finding significant correlation between pronation and MTSS	Studies finding no significant correlation between pronation and MTSS
Rathleff et al., 2012	Bartosik et al., 2010
Raissi et al., 2009	Plisky et al., 2007
Bandholm et al., 2008	Reinking et al., Nov 2007
Reinking et al., Sept 2006	Reinking et al., Jan 2006
Yates et al., 2004	

For full source info, see Craig D. Current developments concerning medial tibial stress syndrome. *Phys Sports Med.* 2009; 37 (4): 1-6.

that study. If each study is similarly designed and well controlled, then you will need to rely on your best judgment—including your own clinical experiences.

Recall that systematic reviews are also available for many clinical treatment options. Thus, if you used PubMed for your regular EBP search and came up with conflicting results, then it would be wise to use the same search parameters in the Cochrane Collaboration Library, where systematic reviews are most plentiful. When research studies come up with conflicting results, many researchers attempt to study the problem further—including using the Cochrane Collaboration. Always remember that systematic reviews may be available for your topic.

A worst-case scenario from your EBP search is that none of your searches turned up anything that was specific to your PICO question. In these instances, which are becoming less and less common, there may simply be no evidence to answer your question. This is when you will need to rely on your own clinical experiences—but with an understanding that what you have been doing previously may not be supported with evidence.

Technology to Remain Current With Evidence

By now, most clinicians are at least aware of new technology that has emerged to assist in updating their evidence-based clinical practice. What we have presented so far in this text has been what we call **pull technology**—meaning that you go into databases and search engines and pull information out to address your clinical question. Conversely, **push technology** consists of **RSS feeds** (Really Simple Syndication), **My NCBI** (through PubMed), **podcasts**, and other digital media that automatically push information to your computer, e-mail inbox, smartphone, or a combination of these. Many research journals, such as the *Journal of Athletic Training*, and professional organizations have RSS feeds that you can request. When you set up RSS feeds or other push technology tools, you request the type of information you want to be updated on as soon as it becomes available. That program then sends a notice whenever a new study has been published on that topic. A word of caution, however: Use RSS feeds judiciously. If you sign up for every RSS feed you come across, you will quickly become overwhelmed.

In addition to push and pull technologies are **apps**. There are many useful apps that you can use on a daily basis in the clinic. Some simply help you take injury evaluation notes, whereas others can provide validity measures for almost every injury evaluation test we use. Early in my schooling, I was taught Apley's compression test to determine the integrity of the knee meniscus. Using an app that reports and routinely updates validity measures of these diagnostic tests, you can find that Apley's compression test has a sensitivity of .22 (meaning that it will be able to detect a true meniscus tear only 22% of the time) and a specificity of .88 (meaning that 88% of all true meniscus tears will test positive with an Apley's test).[4] These sensitivity and specificity scores imply that perhaps we should not be using Apley's compression test to determine injury to the meniscus. These scores can be pulled up within one minute on any smartphone with this type of app.

Foundations of Evidence: Difference Between Specificity and Sensitivity

- SpPin = with high *specificity*, a *positive* test rules *in* the diagnosis
- SnNout = with high *sensitivity*, a *negative* test rules *out* the diagnosis

---

The quick and easy access to many clinical diagnostic and treatment apps has resulted in an explosion in this area of the technology world. From anatomy apps that offer three-dimensional and movable images complete with origins, insertions, innervations, and actions to treatment apps that allow you to make home programs you can print out for specific athletes, the app world is a significant player in the athletic trainer's EBP world. To browse the many apps available, simply get into your app provider and click on Medicine or Medical Apps. From there, you'll be able to browse dozens of tools that may make your clinical practice current and educational for you, your athletes, and your students on a daily basis.

Your Practice Based on Your Clinical Experience

Recall that becoming an evidence-based clinician requires the synthesis of the latest evidence, your clinical experience, and your athlete's values. Whether you are a recently certified athletic trainer or have been in the business for 20-plus years, your own clinical experience is a critical part of this process. Much of what we do clinically comes from what we were taught as students, with adjustments through the years. However, the explosion of published research studies and the immensely improved access to these studies from around the world mean that we may need to replace many of the techniques we learned even five years ago with recently developed techniques that are more effective. Today's students are taught to consider the evidence in all aspects of their clinical practice, even before they become certified.

Some of the skills we perform, whether for injury diagnosis, treatment, or prevention, may have little to no evidence to support them. A prime example is the old method of applying ultrasound for five minutes at 1.2 W/cm^2—regardless of the injury. As a result of new research evidence, athletic trainers now practice much

Table 7.3 Comparison of McMurray Test and Thessaly Test Validity Scores[4]

	Specificity score range	Sensitivity score range
McMurray test	.68-.98; average .77	.16-.87; average .55
Thessaly test	.91-.98; average .96	.66-.90; average .74

more sophisticated, individualized, and effective ultrasound treatments.[5] Many other areas of athletic training practice beyond the obvious modalities provide much evidence to convince us to change how we have historically practiced.

For example, many athletic trainers have historically relied on the McMurray test to determine the integrity of the knee meniscus. This is a difficult test to perform, because you must apply and control four different forces at the knee joint simultaneously while moving the knee and holding the leg with the athlete supine. This has been the gold standard for clinical examination of the knee meniscus for decades. However, more recently, a new test was introduced—the Thessaly test—to evaluate the integrity of the knee meniscus. It is extraordinarily simple to perform and has significantly higher sensitivity and specificity scores than the McMurray test (see table 7.3). However, if you were not staying apprised of the latest research evidence, you may not have heard about this new, better, and easier test. Performing EBP searches and using push technology will allow you to bring your current practice into alignment with that of other evidence-based practitioners. More important, it has great potential to improve the care you provide to your athletes.

Even with the preponderance of research studies available at our desktops, we will still use treatments, tests, and techniques that have not been studied and thus are not supported by evidence. This does not inherently make them wrong, nor does it mean that they don't work. It simply means that they have not been studied. In these instances, you will need to rely on your clinical experience to determine the best course of action for your athletes. For example, although there is little evidence to support any concrete treatment parameters for athletes with MTSS, you may have had good results in decreasing the symptoms by taping athletes' arches. Perhaps you have used this tape in conjunction with soleus muscle stretching before practice and cold whirlpool treatments after practice and found that athletes responded fairly well to this treatment. A lack of research evidence to support a treatment that you have had success with does not mean that you should stop providing that treatment. It usually means that we simply need to do more research. Never underestimate the importance of your own clinical experience. Just remember that if there is evidence about a technique or treatment that can inform your practice, you should update your practice by implementing it.

Your Practice Based on Athlete Preferences and Values

When we ask the athletes we work with exactly what their goal for a specific rehabilitation program is, the most common answer is to get back onto the field, court,

Critical Appraisal of Evidence

In this critical appraisal of evidence, we are evaluating the methods section of a study performed to determine the validity of the Thessaly test for knee meniscus pathology.

Harrison BK, Abell BE, Gibson TW. The Thessaly test for detection of meniscal tears: Validation of a new physical examination technique for primary care medicine. *Clin J Sport Med*. 2009; 19 (1): 9-12.

Study Overview

This was a validation study to determine the clinical usefulness of the new Thessaly test by comparing arthroscopic findings with preoperative clinical examination findings.

Methods

In this study, the authors used 116 patients undergoing knee arthroscopy for suspected meniscal pathology. Prior to the surgery, the Thessaly test was performed on each patient. Findings of the Thessaly test were then compared with findings from the arthroscopy.

Critical Appraisal

1. The results section reported that 65 of the 66 patients with a positive Thessaly test score had arthroscopically verified meniscal tears. The authors do not, however, report what occurred with the other 50 patients. It is assumed that they had negative Thessaly tests, but not explicitly stated.

2. High sensitivity and specificity scores (90.3% and 97.7%, respectively) indicate that the full 116 patients were considered, but just not reported on specific outcomes.

3. A significance level of $p < .001$ indicates a high level of agreement between the Thessaly test and the arthroscopic diagnosis.

4. A negative predictive value of 86.0% indicates that the Thessaly test is capable of ruling out a meniscus tear with fairly good confidence.

or track or into the pool as quickly as possible. They want to quickly and safely return to play. Recent health care research, however, proposes that this goal may not be the only goal that is important to injured athletes.

Most athletic trainers have worked with many athletes who sustain significant season-ending injuries. For a majority of them, depression accompanies their initial injury and commonly well into the rehabilitation work. These athletes have many other concerns beyond returning to play quickly and safely. They may be suffering from a loss of the identity they gain from playing their sport. Perhaps their teammates are talking to them less because they're not on the playing field, causing a sense of alienation. They may be struggling to just get through activities of daily living, but don't know whom to talk to about performing these simple tasks. These common postinjury issues underscore the importance of determining exactly what your athlete's preferences or values are at the outset of postinjury treatment.

The Supreme Importance of Listening

When an athlete comes in to your athletic training room with a new significant injury, it is critical that you give that athlete your full attention not only through the initial injury evaluation and perhaps referral but all the way through the rehabilitation and return to play. This is not possible without the fine-tuned skill of listening. If you are not engaging your athletes with questions about what is troubling them regarding their injuries, their immediate goals and long-term goals, and the most important aspects of how this injury is affecting them currently, then you are not providing the best care possible. Listening to your athletes' concerns, values, and goals will not only inform how you proceed with their care but also make them feel valued and respected.

One of the worst rehabilitation experiences I witnessed was a care provider who, on the first visit post-ACL knee surgery, confirmed the athlete's name and then went to a file cabinet and pulled out the athlete's entire six-month rehabilitation plan. From there, he began to implement day 1. He asked the athlete no questions, took no measurements, and instigated little to no conversation. The athlete reported feeling "faceless" and requested to go elsewhere for rehabilitation. This care provider assumed that all the athlete cared about was returning to play quickly and safely. Therefore, he treated this athlete just like every other postsurgical ACL patient.

Since that era, understanding and addressing athletes' values and needs regarding injury and recovery have garnered significant attention in research and in clinical health care settings everywhere. Subjective athlete-centered questionnaires have been developed to measure athletes' satisfaction with the treatments they have received and with how close they have come to reaching their own goals. The outcome measures include those presented in chapter 2: health-related quality of life, global rating of change, and minimal clinically important difference, to name a few. Numerous electronic tools are also available today for athletes to use to measure and record their life values as associated with their injury and treatment.

To date, electronic questionnaires and surveys have not often been used in athletic training settings. However, we are typically very good at listening to our athletes regarding how they feel they are progressing through rehabilitation programs. The value of electronic questionnaires, however, is that they are robust and easy to administer and truly address the injured athlete's life as a whole—not just around the injured body part. To this end, the best whole-person treatment plan for injured athletes would be to continue to listen to their concerns and goals but also include one of the electronic surveys available to health care clinicians. These tools are discussed further in chapter 8. The benefit of both listening and surveying is increased communication.

Communication

In this third component of evidence-based practice (adjusting your practice based on athletes' values or preferences), communication is key. Always remember that communication is a two-way street. As an athletic trainer, you need to both share information and listen very keenly to your injured athletes. Consider this scenario: A collegiate football player comes to you at practice complaining of feeling dizzy after hitting helmet to helmet with another player. This player suffered and recovered from a concussion two months earlier. After a full evaluation, you determine that it is indeed another concussion, and you refer him to your team physician. After practice, the coach comes in concerned that this athlete is just not tough. The following day, the athlete reports to you that the coach called him the previous evening and told him he was fine and needed to be at practice the following day. The athlete is in his practice uniform but clearly distressed about the pressure from his coach.

In situations such as this, you must take it on yourself to educate the coaches to protect the health and well-being of student-athletes. By listening to this athlete, you learn that he feels significant pressure to not disappoint the coach. This is an important value of many athletes that we must respect and keep in mind when addressing the coach. This does *not* mean that you should change your treatment plan because of the coach's values; rather, you must communicate clearly with the coach to support the athlete. That would be extremely valuable to your athlete. In fact, if you do not do this, the athlete may not report further concussions to you. Thus, understanding what your athlete values is critical to informing the care that you provide.

When considering communication regarding an athlete's injury and treatment, you must communicate both verbally and in writing in a way your athlete can understand. Using common language rather than medical language may be helpful. Your athlete may listen while she's with you but forget home-care instructions by the time she gets home. If she will need help with activities of daily living (e.g., she may not bear weight on a repaired meniscus in her dominant leg for four weeks), communicating daily care instructions in writing will be very helpful. Always check with your athlete in person to make sure she understands any instructions you send home with her. Communication requires listening, respect, and practice. Good communication can help avoid inadequate or ineffective care down the line.

Following are other areas that you should talk with your injured athletes about to learn their preferences or values:

- Potential surgical options and the rehabilitation time lines following those options
- Risks and benefits of various surgical or treatment options
- Insurance boundaries that exist that are important to the athlete
- Financial issues that may affect the athlete, the athlete's family, or both
- Feelings about how the injury may affect daily life and how to address that
- The athlete's immediate and long-term goals of the treatment
- Pressures the athlete feels from coaches, friends, family, teammates, and so on
- Anxieties around the injury and recovery process
- Whether the athlete would like to see a counselor to help with any of these adjustments

Clinical Practice Guidelines

The whole picture of providing evidence-based practice to your athletes includes finding, interpreting, and applying research evidence; considering your own clinical experiences; and communicating thoroughly with your athletes to understand their preferences and values around their recovery. To assist in this process, **clinical practice guidelines (CPGs)** have been developed. The U.S. Department of Health and Human Services' Agency for Healthcare Research and Quality (AHRQ) hosts the National Guideline Clearinghouse (NGC), where CPGs are collected.[6] Clinical practice guidelines incorporate evidence from research, clinical expertise, and athletes' perspectives.

At first glance, CPGs may be difficult to distinguish from systematic reviews. The greatest difference is that CPGs take into account real-time clinical situations presented by clients. The purpose of systematic reviews is to present a summary of research evidence. The purpose of CPGs is to make recommendations for best clinical practice based on the best research evidence, clinical expertise, and athlete perspectives. Specifically, systematic reviews provide a synthesis of the research, whereas CPGs provide best practices in applying that research in clinical situations. Figure 7.1 shows the results of an EBP search for rotator cuff injury management. This is a systematic review, which is at the pinnacle of the evidence pyramid. Using these same search parameters, figure 7.2 provides the results in the form of a CPG for rotator cuff management. Practically speaking, both the systematic review and the CPG can inform your practice. Some athletic trainers prefer to use regular EBP searches to gather initial research articles or systematic reviews, whereas others prefer to use CPGs when available.

Search Resources for CPGs

Clinical practice guidelines are published in peer-reviewed journals, on websites, and in other documents. Some are available through regular EBP search databases or engines, such as PubMed, but these sources do not provide comprehensive, searchable lists of CPGs. To access these comprehensive lists, search in the National Guideline Clearinghouse database (www.guideline.gov; figure 7.3). Additionally, the PEDro database includes some rehabilitation CPGs (figure 7.4). Finally, some organizations maintain CPG lists that target specific professions or groups of users. To date, the National Athletic Trainers' Association website does not maintain a list of CPGs. However, the *Journal of Athletic Training* does publish official position statements, which serve as athletic training–specific clinical practice guidelines. Figure 7.5 shows the result of a search of the *Journal of Athletic Training* site for all position statements.

Practice CPG Search

It's time to perform a CPG search. Consider using the topic of acute low back pain. Using a PICO format, your question might be this: In female field hockey players with acute low back pain, do core strengthening exercises provide greater pain reduction than neural flossing or tension exercises? You may adjust this question however you like to make it more clinically relevant to your current practice.

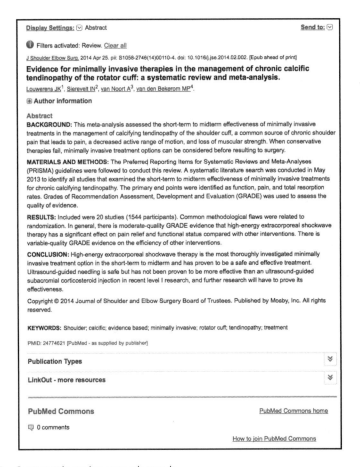

Display Settings: ⊡ Abstract   Send to: ⊡

ⓘ Filters activated: Review. Clear all

J Shoulder Elbow Surg. 2014 Apr 25. pii: S1058-2746(14)00110-4. doi: 10.1016/j.jse.2014.02.002. [Epub ahead of print]

Evidence for minimally invasive therapies in the management of chronic calcific tendinopathy of the rotator cuff: a systematic review and meta-analysis.

Louwerens JK[1], Sierevelt IN[2], van Noort A[3], van den Bekerom MP[4].

⊕ **Author information**

Abstract

BACKGROUND: This meta-analysis assessed the short-term to midterm effectiveness of minimally invasive treatments in the management of calcifying tendinopathy of the shoulder cuff, a common source of chronic shoulder pain that leads to pain, a decreased active range of motion, and loss of muscular strength. When conservative therapies fail, minimally invasive treatment options can be considered before resulting to surgery.

MATERIALS AND METHODS: The Preferred Reporting Items for Systematic Reviews and Meta-Analyses (PRISMA) guidelines were followed to conduct this review. A systematic literature search was conducted in May 2013 to identify all studies that examined the short-term to midterm effectiveness of minimally invasive treatments for chronic calcifying tendinopathy. The primary end points were identified as function, pain, and total resorption rates. Grades of Recommendation Assessment, Development and Evaluation (GRADE) was used to assess the quality of evidence.

RESULTS: Included were 20 studies (1544 participants). Common methodological flaws were related to randomization. In general, there is moderate-quality GRADE evidence that high-energy extracorporeal shockwave therapy has a significant effect on pain relief and functional status compared with other interventions. There is variable-quality GRADE evidence on the efficiency of other interventions.

CONCLUSION: High-energy extracorporeal shockwave therapy is the most thoroughly investigated minimally invasive treatment option in the short-term to midterm and has proven to be a safe and effective treatment. Ultrasound-guided needling is safe but has not been proven to be more effective than an ultrasound-guided subacromial corticosteroid injection in recent level I research, and further research will have to prove its effectiveness.

Copyright © 2014 Journal of Shoulder and Elbow Surgery Board of Trustees. Published by Mosby, Inc. All rights reserved.

KEYWORDS: Shoulder; calcific; evidence based; minimally invasive; rotator cuff; tendinopathy; treatment

PMID: 24774621 [PubMed - as supplied by publisher]

Publication Types   ⊻

LinkOut - more resources   ⊻

PubMed Commons   PubMed Commons home

⊡ 0 comments

                                                How to join PubMed Commons

Figure 7.1 Systematic review search result.
Reprinted from PubMed.gov. Available: www.ncbi.nlm.nih.gov/pubmed.

With your PICO question in hand, search the National Guideline Clearinghouse website (www.guideline.gov), then the PEDro website (www.pedro.fhs.usyd.edu. au), and finally the PubMed website (www.ncbi.nlm.nih.gov/pubmed). Take time to review not only the results but also number of results, ease in reading, and usefulness of each search database regarding the results found. This will help you determine how much time such searches may require and how helpful they may be for your future evidence-based practice.

Practice Altruism

Altruism is the belief in the value of acting for others' good, or selflessness. Applying this to athletic training, altruism may be defined as the belief in the value of providing care solely to promote the health and well-being of our athletes. This is one of the many tenets that our great profession was founded on. We cannot act altruistically if we are not keeping up with the enormous amount of research that is being produced and is readily available in the health care professions in this

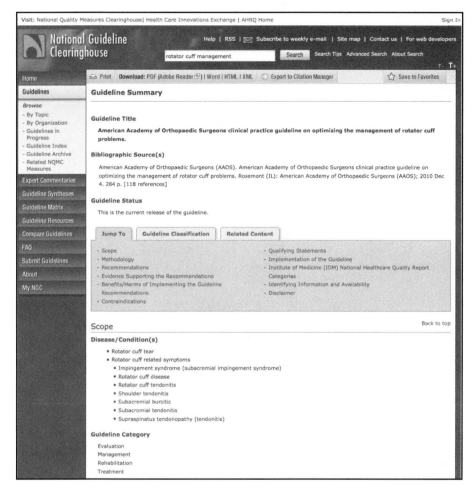

Figure 7.2 CPG search result.

Reprinted from Agency for Healthcare Research and Quality 2014.

age of evidence-based practice. By having clinical practices that are infused with evidence-based skills, we assure our athletes that we are current and providing them with the best care possible.

Practicing altruism requires us to give of ourselves for the good of our athletes. This can become draining and lead to burnout in any health care profession. To avoid this, we must be certain that we are making time for ourselves outside of work. If we do not create a work–life boundary, then practicing altruism can become very difficult. It is hard to give to others when we are drained. But when we fail to practice altruistically, we fail to provide the best medical care possible. The primacy of our athletes' health must always remain front and center. Thus, practicing altruism requires us to both put more effort into our clinical lives by practicing EBP (to keep current) and to set strong boundaries to ensure that we are "filling our tanks" with life outside of our athletic training work. This allows us to provide the best care possible to our athletes and to have the energy to do so at all times.

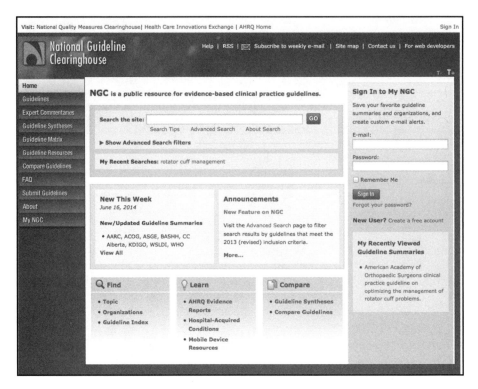

Figure 7.3 Initial search page on National Guideline Clearinghouse.
Reprinted from Agency for Healthcare Research and Quality 2014.

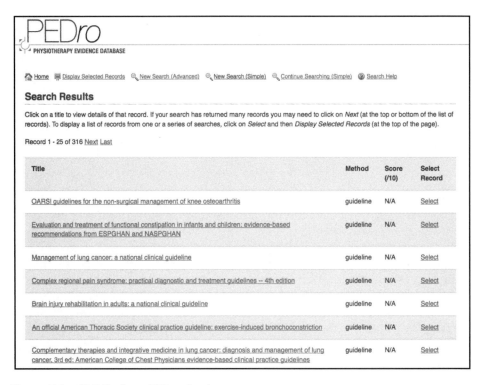

Figure 7.4 CPG list from PEDro database.
Reprinted from PEDro.org. Available: www.pedro.org.au/wp-content/uploads/PEDro_scale.pdf.

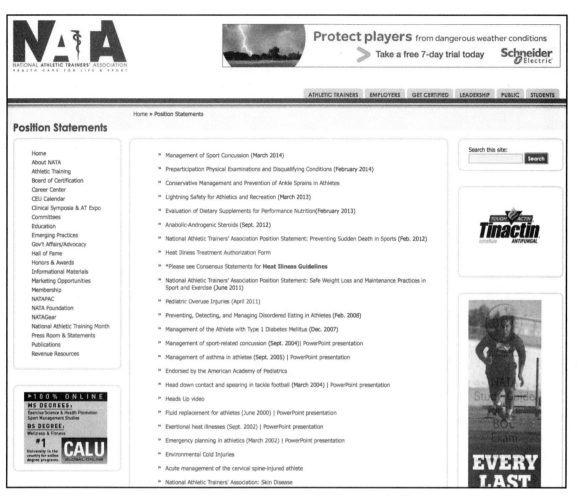

Figure 7.5 Output from *Journal of Athletic Training* search for position statements.
Reprinted from www.journalofathletictraining.org.

Consider this scenario: A collegiate men's basketball player sustains a severely broken nose in a Friday night game. Because he's the starting center, he is referred to an ear, nose, and throat (ENT) physician immediately that evening. The physician says that it would not harm the broken bones any further for the athlete to play in the game the next evening, but he must wear a solid, full-face, clear mask so that a direct blow to the face is not absorbed by the nose area. The next morning, the coach and everyone else are so anxious about creating a face mask in time for the game that no one stops to ask the athlete how he's feeling. When the athletic trainer finally does, the athlete reports feeling like a token on a chess board that no one really cares about—they just want him on the court. Further, he reports not being able to breathe well, and blood is periodically running down the back of his throat. In further conversation, the athletic trainer finds out that the athlete does not believe he can play and contribute in any meaningful way to the team that evening.

With this information, the athletic trainer has two options. The first is to tell the athlete that he needs to get on the court with the face mask that evening and see how it goes. This option may appease the coach and perhaps others above the coach if it's a critical game for the team, but it does not support the athlete. The second option is to listen to the athlete's concerns and values and then to support his well-being by having him sit out the game.

In our role as athletic trainers, we are put in situations like this far more often than most people realize. When this happens, we must be certain that we are current with the latest evidence on the situation and that our decision should be in the best interest of the athlete. It is the coaches' job to win. It is our job to ensure the well-being of injured athletes. If we do not do this, no one else will. We must practice altruism by keeping current with EBP, maintaining a work–life balance, and always protecting and supporting our athletes' health and well-being.

Summary

This chapter provided tools and suggestions for infusing your current daily clinical practice with EBP skills based on evidence, your previous clinical experiences, and your athletes' values. Whereas the previous chapters explained how to find and appraise evidence, this chapter focused on how to incorporate the skills you discover into your daily routine, despite common barriers. Push technologies, pull technologies, and apps were discussed and related to your daily practice through several clinical examples. Clinical practice guidelines (CPGs) were introduced as a new evidence tool, along with search techniques for finding them. Finally, the importance of being altruistic when implementing EBP into your daily routine to ensure the well-being of your athletes was emphasized.

References

1. Hankemeier D, Van Lunen B. Perceptions of approved clinical instructors: Barriers in the implementation of evidence-based practice. *J Athl Train*. 2013; 48 (3): 382-393.

2. Fetters LK, Tilson J. *Evidence based physical therapy*. Philadelphia: Davis; 2012.

3. Welch C, Hankemeier D, Wyant A, Hays D, Pitney W, Van Lunen B. Future directions of evidence-based practice in athletic training: Perceived strategies. *J Athl Train*. 2014; 49 (2): 234-244.

4. Clinically Relevant Technologies. Clinical orthopedic exam (CORE) application. CRTech, LLC [Medical Apps]. 2012.

5. Draper D. Free communications: Emerging interventions for thermal and iontophoresis treatment. *J Athl Train*. 2014; 49 (3 supp): 45-48.

6. U.S. Department of Health and Human Services. Agency for Healthcare Research and Quality. Clinical practice guidelines. National Guideline Clearinghouse website. www.guideline.gov. Accessed May 15, 2014.

Overview of Outcome Measures

Outcome measures have garnered much attention in health care research since the early 2000s. Indeed, they are what produce answers on which to base evidence-based practice decisions. Choosing the outcome measures that will improve your clinical practice and ultimately injured athlete outcomes is a key component in becoming a competent evidence-based clinician. This chapter describes types of outcome measures, their psychometric properties, and how to use them to improve your clinical practice. Understanding outcome measures is key to understanding the evidence.

Types of Outcome Measures

Outcome measures are generally categorized as either performance measures or questionnaires (surveys). An **outcome measure** is any characteristic measured to assess how an athlete is progressing or feeling in the moment.[1,2] Commonly, outcome measures are assessed at the beginning of a rehabilitation program, midway through the program, and when the athlete returns to full competition or is otherwise discharged. Finding an appropriate outcome measure for a specific condition can be difficult. For example, Chapman and colleagues performed a review of common outcome measures of treatment success for chronic low back pain.[3] After inclusion and exclusion criteria were applied, they found 75 measures cited to evaluate chronic low back pain. Their recommendation was to first consider

Table 8.1 Common Outcome Measures in Rehabilitation Settings

Name	Type	Topic of measure
Modified Oswestry Low Back Disability Questionnaire	Questionnaire	Effect of low back pain on daily life
Standardized concussion tests	Performance measures	Performance effects of concussion
Focus on Therapeutic Outcomes tool	Questionnaire	Effect of injury on daily life
Range of motion, strength, girth, and proprioception tests	Performance measures	Physical effects of injury

outcome measures that were reliable, valid, and responsive to change. We delve into these properties later in the chapter. Table 8.1 offers some common outcome measures used in rehabilitation settings.

Questionnaires

Questionnaires are completed by athletes typically before, during, and at the end of rehabilitation after injury or illness. They include questions about the athlete's confidence in performing certain tasks, such as sitting for a long time, walking, running, climbing stairs, and lifting heavy items. Athletes report their level of ability or comfort in performing each task on a graded scale. Other questions might address how well they're sleeping at night, whether medications help their condition, whether their condition is causing any depression or social angst, and how well they perform activities of daily living.

The field of athletic training has not historically used questionnaires. However, their availability on various electronic platforms for mobile devices now makes it easy to use these valuable tools to determine not only athletes' progress but how they are feeling about their progress. This can help us address quality of life measures for injured athletes, which have gone largely ignored in the past.

Performance Measures

Performance measures have been used to gauge the status of injured athletes since the beginning of our profession. For example, for an athlete who has had knee surgery, we typically take girth and range of motion measurements on the first visit after surgery and compare those with measurements of the unaffected limb. After we progress the athlete to a moderate level of functionality, we reassess those measures and compare them to day 1 measures to quantify progress. Finally, when the athlete is ready to return to play, we repeat those measures once more (along with sport-specific physical tests) to determine whether she has returned to normal measures when compared bilaterally.

When you find performance outcome measures in the literature, they are typically for balance, memory, or a return to normal function during activities of daily living rather than for athletic performance. For athletic trainers in rehabilitation clinics or hospital settings, such outcome measures are normal practice. Regardless of the setting, whatever goals your athlete has set should be measured with performance outcome measures before, during, and at the end of rehabilitation.

Ideally, rehabilitation programs in all athletic training settings would use both types of outcome measures.

Psychometric Properties of Outcome Measures

The usefulness of an outcome measure should be evaluated on three **psychometric properties** (the intrinsic properties of an outcome measure): (1) the reliability of the measure (Are the results reproducible?), (2) the validity of the measure (Does the instrument assess what it is supposed to assess?), and (3) the clinical meaningfulness of the measure (Does this outcome matter to the athlete?).

Foundations of Evidence: Psychometric Properties of Outcome Measures

- Reliability—Are the results reproducible?
- Validity—Does the instrument assess what it is intended to assess?
- Clinical meaningfulness—Does this outcome matter to the athlete?

Determining the Reliability of Outcome Measures

When any instrument (e.g., a questionnaire) or equipment (e.g., a body fat measuring tool) is used in a research study, its reliability must be tested and reported. Reliability is the ability of an instrument, tool, or person to produce consistent results if measuring the same subject again and again. The four most common types of reliability measures are intrarater (person reliability), interrater (person reliability), test–retest (instrument reliability), and internal consistency (instrument reliability).[4] These are reviewed in chapter 3.

When choosing an outcome measure to use with an athlete, be sure to find the reliability measures reported in the literature. Internal consistency is commonly used for surveys and questionnaires. These scores demonstrate intraclass correlation (ICC) using a Cronbach's alpha score. The ideal Cronbach's alpha score, one that indicates a reliable instrument, should range from .75 to 1.0.[4]

For example, to assess an athlete's sense of ankle stability, you may consider using the Foot and Ankle Outcome Score (FAOS) instrument. This instrument has been tested for reliability and validity numerous times and adapted to various cultures around the world. Thus, when you perform an EBP search to find the reliability of the FAOS, you will find scores for adaptations in various countries. The FAOS adaptation for the Dutch version was reported to have a Cronbach's alpha score of .90 to .96, demonstrating excellent internal consistency reliability (figure 8.1).[5] This indicates that this instrument would be a reliable choice for determining your athlete's sense of ankle stability at the beginning of the rehabilitation program, at the midpoint, and at return to play.

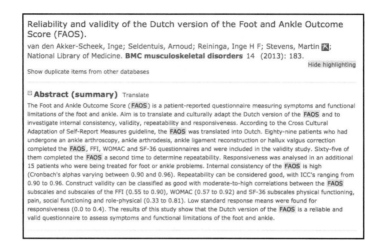

Reliability and validity of the Dutch version of the Foot and Ankle Outcome Score (FAOS).

van den Akker-Scheek, Inge; Seldentuis, Arnoud; Reininga, Inge H F; Stevens, Martin ⬛;
National Library of Medicine. **BMC musculoskeletal disorders** 14 (2013): 183.

Hide highlighting

Show duplicate items from other databases

⊟ **Abstract (summary)** Translate

The Foot and Ankle Outcome Score (FAOS) is a patient-reported questionnaire measuring symptoms and functional limitations of the foot and ankle. Aim is to translate and culturally adapt the Dutch version of the FAOS and to investigate internal consistency, validity, repeatability and responsiveness. According to the Cross Cultural Adaptation of Self-Report Measures guideline, the FAOS was translated into Dutch. Eighty-nine patients who had undergone an ankle arthroscopy, ankle arthrodesis, ankle ligament reconstruction or hallux valgus correction completed the FAOS, FFI, WOMAC and SF-36 questionnaires and were included in the validity study. Sixty-five of them completed the FAOS a second time to determine repeatability. Responsiveness was analysed in an additional 15 patients who were being treated for foot or ankle problems. Internal consistency of the FAOS is high (Cronbach's alphas varying between 0.90 and 0.96). Repeatability can be considered good, with ICC's ranging from 0.90 to 0.96. Construct validity can be classified as good with moderate-to-high correlations between the FAOS subscales and subscales of the FFI (0.55 to 0.90), WOMAC (0.57 to 0.92) and SF-36 subscales physical functioning, pain, social functioning and role-physical (0.33 to 0.81). Low standard response means were found for responsiveness (0.0 to 0.4). The results of this study show that the Dutch version of the FAOS is a reliable and valid questionnaire to assess symptoms and functional limitations of the foot and ankle.

Figure 8.1 Article reporting reliability and validity scores for the FAOS outcome instrument.
Reprinted from proquest.com.

Determining the Validity of Outcome Measures

Validity addresses how well an instrument, tool, or full study measures what it is intended to measure.[4] For example, the FAOS would not be a valid instrument to use with an athlete who has a knee injury; it is intended to assess the foot or ankle. The three general types of validity are content validity (including face validity and expert panel evaluation), criterion validity (comparing one tool to a gold standard tool; includes concurrent and predictive validity), and construct validity (the most rigorous validity measure; includes known-groups, convergent, and discriminant validity). These are reviewed in chapter 3.

As with reliability, when choosing an outcome measure for a clinical situation, you need to be certain that the instrument has been validated in the literature. Most often, studies that report reliability scores also report validity scores. The statistical measure used to report validity is the Pearson's or Spearman's rho correlation, which you will see reported as an *r* value.[4] Correlations close to 0.0 indicate no correlation between the constructs. Scores closer to +1.0 indicate a strong **positive correlation** between constructs, whereas scores closer to −1.0 indicate a strong **negative correlation** (i.e., when one construct score increases, the other construct score decreases).[4]

Consider an athlete who is comparing his sense of knee instability when walking with the degree of anterior translation of his tibia during an anterior cruciate ligament integrity test. As the amount of anterior translation increases, his sense of instability should increase. This reflects a positive correlation. An athlete who has suffered a rotator cuff injury may be comparing pain with external rotation of the glenohumeral joint with her external rotation range of motion. As expected, as her pain scores decrease, her range of motion measures increase. This is an example of negative correlation.

Thus, validity scores, whether negative or positive, indicate how helpful the measure would be in your evidence-based practice. Validity scores closer to zero indicate that the outcome measure is less valid for the purpose intended.

Determining the Clinical Meaningfulness of Outcome Measures

With reliability and validity measure scores in hand, you are ready to consider the third component of outcome measure appropriateness for your clinical practice—its clinical meaningfulness. **Clinical meaningfulness** is an outcome measure's ability to provide measures of change in the athlete's condition that are valuable to the athlete and the clinician.[1,6,7] The two most common measures used to quantify clinical meaningfulness are minimal detectible change (MDC) and minimal clinically important difference (MCID). These are discussed in chapter 2.

MDC is the amount of change needed to exceed a natural variation and represent true change in the athlete's recovery. Most commonly, MDC is measured using a high-quality methodology that is specific to a certain population and has test–retest reliability. Figure 8.2 demonstrates such a study for MDC in quadriceps strength for athletes with knee osteoarthritis.[8] You can see that isometric and isokinetic quadriceps strength scores (which are necessary for denoting a minimal detectable change) are reported as 25.02 Nm and 33.90 Nm, respectively, for this population. The test–retest reliability scores are reported as ICCs of .93 to .98. Thus, this is considered a very reliable measure. Further, the authors report an MDC score for the percentage of voluntary activation as 6.6%, which means that a change of 6.6% of voluntary quadriceps activation is the minimal detectable change increase necessary to represent true change in the athlete's recovery. Thus, for your athletes with knee osteoarthritis, this study may provide quantifiable measures of quadriceps strength improvement to use as goals during the rehabilitation process.

MCID is the amount of change necessary in an outcome measure to be meaningful to the athlete and signify that it is time for a change in care or a progression to the next phase in rehabilitation. This should be an athlete-identified change, whenever possible. This measure may also be reported as MID, or minimal important

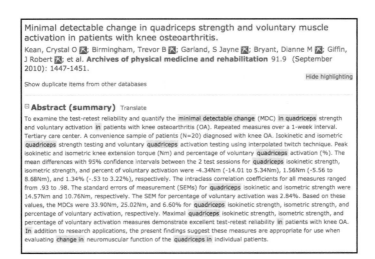

Minimal detectable change in quadriceps strength and voluntary muscle activation in patients with knee osteoarthritis.

Kean, Crystal O ⊠; Birmingham, Trevor B ⊠; Garland, S Jayne ⊠; Bryant, Dianne M ⊠; Giffin, J Robert ⊠; et al. **Archives of physical medicine and rehabilitation** 91.9 (September 2010): 1447-1451.

Show duplicate items from other databases

Hide highlighting

⊟ **Abstract (summary)** Translate

To examine the test-retest reliability and quantify the minimal detectable change (MDC) in quadriceps strength and voluntary activation in patients with knee osteoarthritis (OA). Repeated measures over a 1-week interval. Tertiary care center. A convenience sample of patients (N=20) diagnosed with knee OA. Isokinetic and isometric quadriceps strength testing and voluntary quadriceps activation testing using interpolated twitch technique. Peak isokinetic and isometric knee extension torque (Nm) and percentage of voluntary quadriceps activation (%). The mean differences with 95% confidence intervals between the 2 test sessions for quadriceps isokinetic strength, isometric strength, and percent of voluntary activation were -4.34Nm (-14.01 to 5.34Nm), 1.56Nm (-5.56 to 8.68Nm), and 1.34% (-.53 to 3.22%), respectively. The intraclass correlation coefficients for all measures ranged from .93 to .98. The standard errors of measurement (SEMs) for quadriceps isokinetic and isometric strength were 14.57Nm and 10.76Nm, respectively. The SEM for percentage of voluntary activation was 2.84%. Based on these values, the MDCs were 33.90Nm, 25.02Nm, and 6.60% for quadriceps isokinetic strength, isometric strength, and percentage of voluntary activation, respectively. Maximal quadriceps isokinetic strength, isometric strength, and percentage of voluntary activation measures demonstrate excellent test-retest reliability in patients with knee OA. In addition to research applications, the present findings suggest these measures are appropriate for use when evaluating change in neuromuscular function of the quadriceps in individual patients.

Figure 8.2 A study to establish MDC in quadriceps strength for athletes with knee osteoarthritis.

Reprinted from proquest.com.

difference. The athlete reports the amount of change that would be significant to him, often on a sliding functional outcome scale. For outcome measures that report MCIDs, those MCIDs are typically specific to a defined population. MCID scores are different for different outcome measures.

Figure 8.3 shows MCID scores for two shoulder pain and functional outcome measures for athletes with rotator cuff injury who were treated nonsurgically.[9] A total of 81 athletes took an initial test and the same test six weeks into their rehabilitation. A 2-point change for the outcome measure of the Simple Shoulder Test (SST) and a 12- to 17-point change for the outcome measure of the American Shoulder and Elbow Surgeons (ASES) were determined to be the MCID for the athletes in that population. When working with athletes being treated nonsurgically for rotator cuff injury, you could use either of these outcome measure tools (the SST or ASES) knowing that a change in your athlete's scores of 2 for the SST or greater than 12 for the ASES would denote a favorable MCID. Such scores may indicate that the athlete is ready to progress to the next phase of rehabilitation. If these scores are not reached after six weeks of rehabilitation, a change may be needed in treatment parameters or you may need to address any shortcomings in your treatment. After choosing an outcome reporting tool or measure, see whether MCID scores are available.

The relationship between MDC and MCID is important to understand. The minimal detectable change takes into account the natural variability of the outcome measure and should always be a lower score than the minimal clinically important difference. If the MCID is lower, the variance of the MDC is likely too great and would cloud your ability to detect clinically meaningful change. Remember that the MDC is a minimal *detectable* change. This means that a change is present, but the athlete may not interpret that change as important or meaningful. If one of your athletes is prescribed an anti-inflammatory drug for an injury, the drug may be

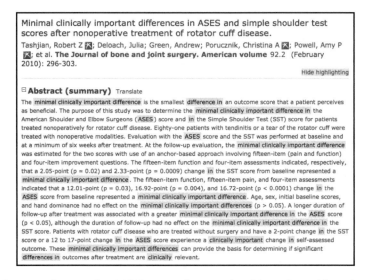

Minimal clinically important differences in ASES and simple shoulder test scores after nonoperative treatment of rotator cuff disease.

Tashjian, Robert Z [X]; Deloach, Julia; Green, Andrew; Porucznik, Christina A [X]; Powell, Amy P [X]; et al. **The Journal of bone and joint surgery. American volume** 92.2 (February 2010): 296-303.

Hide highlighting

□ **Abstract (summary)** Translate

The minimal clinically important difference is the smallest difference in an outcome score that a patient perceives as beneficial. The purpose of this study was to determine the minimal clinically important difference in the American Shoulder and Elbow Surgeons (ASES) score and in the Simple Shoulder Test (SST) score for patients treated nonoperatively for rotator cuff disease. Eighty-one patients with tendinitis or a tear of the rotator cuff were treated with nonoperative modalities. Evaluation with the ASES score and the SST was performed at baseline and at a minimum of six weeks after treatment. At the follow-up evaluation, the minimal clinically important difference was estimated for the two scores with use of an anchor-based approach involving fifteen-item (pain and function) and four-item improvement questions. The fifteen-item function and four-item assessments indicated, respectively, that a 2.05-point (p = 0.02) and 2.33-point (p = 0.0009) change in the SST score from baseline represented a minimal clinically important difference. The fifteen-item function, fifteen-item pain, and four-item assessments indicated that a 12.01-point (p = 0.03), 16.92-point (p = 0.004), and 16.72-point (p < 0.0001) change in the ASES score from baseline represented a minimal clinically important difference. Age, sex, initial baseline scores, and hand dominance had no effect on the minimal clinically important differences (p > 0.05). A longer duration of follow-up after treatment was associated with a greater minimal clinically important difference in the ASES score (p < 0.05), although the duration of follow-up had no effect on the minimal clinically important difference in the SST score. Patients with rotator cuff disease who are treated without surgery and have a 2-point change in the SST score or a 12 to 17-point change in the ASES score experience a clinically important change in self-assessed outcome. These minimal clinically important differences can provide the basis for determining if significant differences in outcomes after treatment are clinically relevant.

Figure 8.3 A study reporting MCID scores for two shoulder pain and function outcome measures for athletes with nonsurgical rotator cuff injury.

Reprinted from proquest.com.

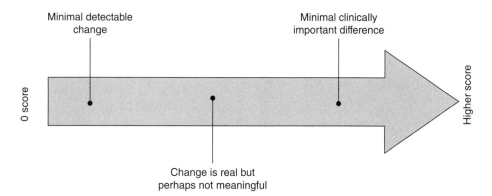

Figure 8.4 The relationship between MDC and MCID scores of clinical meaningfulness.

detected in her bloodstream 30 minutes after taking the first dose (the theoretical MDC). However, the athlete would not report an important difference until her injured limb began to feel better (the theoretical MCID), which may not occur until several doses later. Figure 8.4 illustrates the relationship between the MDC and the MCID outcome measures of clinical meaningfulness.

Communicating Outcomes

We have all worked with athletes who have come back from physicians' appointments with vague (at best) injury diagnosis reports or rehabilitation instructions. Working with athletes to establish clear and helpful communication patterns is one of the challenges we face regarding all facets of athletic health care. Communication in the athletic training room requires excellent listening skills, clear and concise writing skills, and thorough verbal skills. The importance of excellent listening skills was addressed in chapter 7. This section focuses on the written and verbal communication of treatment outcomes with athletes and other members of the sports medicine team.

Communicating Outcomes to the Athlete

Whether you are using questionnaire or survey outcome measures or performance outcome measures, you need to communicate what the measures are assessing, why that is important, and how those measures will inform the athlete's progress through the rehabilitation program. The better informed your athletes are, the more they will understand what is happening to them and why, which fosters motivation and compliance with the rehabilitation program.

For example, we often take strength, girth, and range of motion measurements periodically throughout a rehabilitation program. At times, we do so to assess the athlete's progress. At other times, we do so to provide motivation, perhaps in the form of positive feedback regarding how hard he has worked to gain more range of motion. This is an example of using performance outcome measures and communicating them to the athlete to gain his trust and motivate him to keep working hard in the program. If we take the measurements and do not communicate them to the athlete, we fall short of realizing their full benefit.

Let's say you have decided to have your athlete fill out a questionnaire that assesses the effects of her injury on her daily life three times in the rehabilitation process: prior to rehabilitation, midway through the program, and after return to play. Recall that questionnaires can inform you of your athlete's values, which you should consider when making evidence-based practice decisions. To gain your athlete's trust, you should take the time to verbally describe the questionnaire, what it is assessing, and why it is important (e.g., to help you choose exercises to prescribe or to help her establish her own rehabilitation goals). This is far better than just handing her the questionnaire, waiting while she fills it out, and then setting it on a desk before starting the physical examination. Too often, athletic trainers assume that athletes are concerned only with getting back to participation. The reality is that often they have other concerns that you will discover only by engaging in thorough communication.

When communicating with your athletes, use terms they understand. Some athletes have a good understanding of health and medical terminology; others do not. Thus, it is important to consistently ask your athletes if they understand what you've been talking about or what you've just written for them. All athletes have the right to know what's going on with their bodies, so take the time to double- and triple-check that they understand the care you are providing. Use simple medical terms when possible, and be concise with the information you provide. Provide enough information to be clear but not so much that the athlete becomes overwhelmed. Visual aids such as pictures, drawings, and videos generally improve the athlete's understanding a great deal.

Communicating Outcomes to the Sports Medicine Team

Given the array of health care specialists that make up the sports medicine team, communication regarding specific athletes and their progress is critical for the delivery of efficient and effective care. In the United States, this communication must follow **HIPAA** (Health Insurance Portability and Accountability Act) regulations, as with all medical record management by health care professionals. (For further HIPAA information, visit the federal government website.) It is important to limit the sharing of athlete medical information as much as possible while still promoting effective care. If an outcome measure will inform another member of the sports medicine team regarding the care he is providing to the same athlete, then you should communicate that outcome measure within HIPAA guidelines. Electronic medical records (EMR) make the sharing of information much easier than previously, but make sure you are following HIPAA regulations to ensure the medical confidentiality of your athletes. EMRs, X-ray results, MRI results, blood test results, and so on can be shared quickly among medical professionals even when they are in different states or countries.

For example, if your postsurgical athlete is progressing faster through her rehabilitation program than you expected, you should communicate this to her physician. This communication would usually include performance outcome measures such as gains in strength and range of motion. However, in this situation, the team psychologist would likely not need to know these outcome measures. Limiting the information you share and the people you share it with is as important as making sure all of the right team members have the information they need to progress the care of each athlete.

Assessing Your Practice

The obvious purpose of outcome measures is to determine whether the care is benefiting the athlete. Although providing care is in your job description, evaluating the outcomes of that care is commonly not. However, to be confident that you are providing the best care possible, you must be an evidence-based practitioner. The first several chapters of this text provide methods for finding and assessing the evidence. Chapter 7 explains how to use the evidence you find in your daily practice. This chapter addresses using outcome measures to determine whether the evidence-based care you are providing is helping your athlete. Reflecting on each of these areas encompasses the assessment of your practice.

Using EBP Skills Consistently

Recall from chapter 7 that common barriers to becoming an evidence-based athletic trainer include a lack of time, equipment and literature access, research and statistics knowledge, search and appraisal skills, and generalizability of the research to your athletic populations.[10] In addition to identifying these barriers, we offered several solutions: seeking more EBP resources, gaining access to more preappraised resources (such as CATs and systematic reviews), attending EBP-specific workshops, engaging in peer discussions and mentorship regarding EBP, and gaining more experience simply by performing repetitive EBP searches until you are comfortable with the process.[11]

One of the most difficult parts of implementing any new large change is taking the first step. Whether this is in your personal life (e.g., exercising more) or in your professional life (e.g., performing EBP searches three times a week), it takes dedication to change. This is why we have suggested that you perform EBP searches and appraisals throughout the text. To make the necessary change in our profession and in your own clinical practice, write time into your calendar to perform three searches this week (roughly 30 to 60 minutes for each search).

Perhaps you feel most comfortable using PubMed for your EBP searches. Perhaps you find the systematic reviews in the Cochrane Collaboration more immediately helpful. Or perhaps you've decided to have each of your injured athletes complete a standard quality of life questionnaire to assess their values and progress throughout the rehabilitation program. Whatever the case, infusing your daily practice with EBP skills is important to your athletes, to your practice, and to our profession. Consistency in implementing these EBP skills is key.

Being Satisfied With the Outcomes

Once you begin to implement EBP on a daily basis, pay attention to any changes in the outcomes. Are your athletes recovering faster? Do they have fewer reinjuries? Are you understanding more about their values, beyond how soon they can return to play? Have you discovered information or evidence that has changed your treatment or evaluation of certain injuries dramatically? Perhaps you've discovered evidence that has made your daily practice more efficient. These are just some of the things that can occur through EBP.

To measure your athletes' satisfaction with the care you are providing, you can use a quality of life survey, global rating of change survey, or any other psychometrically sound outcome instrument. You may also consider asking some of your return customers if they have noticed a difference in their own satisfaction from before you began using EBP skills. Measuring your satisfaction with your new EBP skills usually requires reflecting on your pre-EBP practices and comparing them with your current EBP practices. Continual learning is one of the greatest benefits of implementing EBP into your daily practice.

Finding and Using Psychometrically Sound Outcome Instruments

Recall the three psychometric properties used to assess outcome measures: reliability, validity, and clinical meaningfulness. When searching for an outcome instrument, make sure each of these properties is clearly reported in studies assessing the quality of the instrument. Some outcome measure instruments are used to assess physical changes, such as range of motion, strength, or pain levels, whereas others are used to assess the athlete's sense of progress toward reaching the goals of the rehabilitation program. Finding the right instrument for a particular purpose requires the same EBP search techniques as finding the right evidence to most effectively assess or treat a specific injury.

To begin your search, be clear about the type of outcome measure you are seeking (e.g., a questionnaire to assess the impact of the injury on the athlete's life, or a physical outcome measure, such as the ImPACT test, to assess the degree of the injury). With this in mind, go to PubMed and enter your search terms. Those terms may include some of, or any combination of, the following: *orthopedic, outcome measure, quality of life, MCID, MDC, functional assessment, pain rating scale*. If you search for *orthopedic outcome measure* and receive over a thousand results, you can pare down the search from there by adding qualifiers, such as a specific body part or whether you are looking for a functional or pain-related outcome measure. Take the time now to perform such a search, perhaps for a functional outcome measure for baseball players who have injured the rotator cuff.

With the results from your search, you should be able to find research articles that clearly report the psychometric properties of the outcome measures you found. Commonly, the reliability and validity of an outcome measure are reported in the same research article (see figure 8.1). Once you find an outcome measure with good reliability and validity scores, you can search the evidence again for clinical meaningfulness studies that report MCID or MDC statistics. Figure 8.5 shows the results from using this secondary search technique from the same initial search used to produce figure 8.1.[12]

The same search techniques can be used to find an outcome measure that assesses the impact of the injury on the athlete's daily life. Many of these instruments are available to clinicians, usually in the form of online tools. Several health care professions are beginning to increase the use of these instruments to determine the quality of the care provided by practitioners. Indeed, the future may require athletic trainers to do the same. These tools can demonstrate change, from the athlete's perspective, regarding both function and satisfaction relative to the care provided. Insurance companies are also beginning to invest in these types of outcome measures. Figure 8.6 offers a simple global rating of change scale.[13] Figure 8.7 shows a more complex questionnaire, the Knee Injury and Osteoarthritis

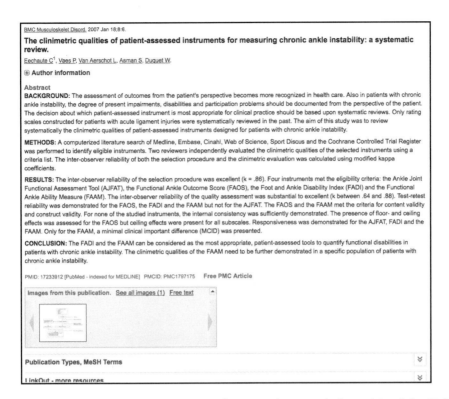

BMC Musculoskelet Disord. 2007 Jan 18;8:6.

The clinimetric qualities of patient-assessed instruments for measuring chronic ankle instability: a systematic review.

Eechaute C[1], Vaes P, Van Aerschot L, Asman S, Duquet W.

⊕ Author information

Abstract

BACKGROUND: The assessment of outcomes from the patient's perspective becomes more recognized in health care. Also in patients with chronic ankle instability, the degree of present impairments, disabilities and participation problems should be documented from the perspective of the patient. The decision about which patient-assessed instrument is most appropriate for clinical practice should be based upon systematic reviews. Only rating scales constructed for patients with acute ligament injuries were systematically reviewed in the past. The aim of this study was to review systematically the clinimetric qualities of patient-assessed instruments designed for patients with chronic ankle instability.

METHODS: A computerized literature search of Medline, Embase, Cinahl, Web of Science, Sport Discus and the Cochrane Controlled Trial Register was performed to identify eligible instruments. Two reviewers independently evaluated the clinimetric qualities of the selected instruments using a criteria list. The inter-observer reliability of both the selection procedure and the clinimetric evaluation was calculated using modified kappa coefficients.

RESULTS: The inter-observer reliability of the selection procedure was excellent (k = .86). Four instruments met the eligibility criteria: the Ankle Joint Functional Assessment Tool (AJFAT), the Functional Ankle Outcome Score (FAOS), the Foot and Ankle Disability Index (FADI) and the Functional Ankle Ability Measure (FAAM). The inter-observer reliability of the quality assessment was substantial to excellent (k between .64 and .88). Test-retest reliability was demonstrated for the FAOS, the FADI and the FAAM but not for the AJFAT. The FAOS and the FAAM met the criteria for content validity and construct validity. For none of the studied instruments, the internal consistency was sufficiently demonstrated. The presence of floor- and ceiling effects was assessed for the FAOS but ceiling effects were present for all subscales. Responsiveness was demonstrated for the AJFAT, FADI and the FAAM. Only for the FAAM, a minimal clinical important difference (MCID) was presented.

CONCLUSION: The FADI and the FAAM can be considered as the most appropriate, patient-assessed tools to quantify functional disabilities in patients with chronic ankle instability. The clinimetric qualities of the FAAM need to be further demonstrated in a specific population of patients with chronic ankle instability.

PMID: 17233912 [PubMed - indexed for MEDLINE] PMCID: PMC1797175 **Free PMC Article**

Images from this publication. See all images (1) Free text

Publication Types, MeSH Terms ⯆

LinkOut - more resources ⯆

Figure 8.5 Article reporting the results of a secondary search for MCID of the FAOS outcome instrument after a previous search for reliability and validity scores for the FAOS.
Reprinted from PubMed.gov. Available: www.ncbi.nlm.nih.gov/pubmed.

Thank you for the opportunity to assist in your rehabilitation. The following rating scale allows us to review the overall outcome of your condition with physical therapy intervention. It allows us to review your physical therapy outcome, which helps guide our treatment to better serve our patients in the future. The Global Rating of Change (GROC) has been well documented and extensively used in research as an outcome measure as well as to compare outcome measures.

Please rate the overall condition of your injured body part or region *from the time that you began treatment until now.* Check only one:

A very great deal worse	(-7)	About the same	(0)	A very great deal better	(7)
A great deal worse	(-6)			A great deal better	(6)
Quite a bit worse	(-5)			Quite a bit better	(5)
Moderately worse	(-4)			Moderately better	(4)
Somewhat worse	(-3)			Somewhat better	(3)
A little bit worse	(-2)			A little bit better	(2)
A tiny bit worse	(-1)			A tiny bit better	(1)

Figure 8.6 A simple global rating of change scale.
Reprinted from Cisco LifeConnections and Stanford Health Care.

KOOS Knee Survey

Today's date: _____   Date of birth: _____

Name: _____

Instructions

This survey asks for your view about your knee. This information will help us keep track of how you feel about your knee and how well you are able to perform your usual activities. Answer every question by ticking the appropriate box, only one box for each question. If you are unsure about how to answer a question, please give the best answer you can.

Symptoms

These questions should be answered thinking of your knee symptoms during the last week.

S1. Do you have swelling in your knee?

☐ Never   ☐ Rarely   ☐ Sometimes   ☐ Often   ☐ Always

S2. Do you feel grinding, hear clicking or any other type of noise when your knee moves?

☐ Never   ☐ Rarely   ☐ Sometimes   ☐ Often   ☐ Always

S3. Does your knee catch or hang up when moving?

☐ Never   ☐ Rarely   ☐ Sometimes   ☐ Often   ☐ Always

S4. Can you straighten your knee fully?

☐ Never   ☐ Rarely   ☐ Sometimes   ☐ Often   ☐ Always

S5. Can you bend your knee fully?

☐ Never   ☐ Rarely   ☐ Sometimes   ☐ Often   ☐ Always

Stiffness

The following questions concern the amount of joint stiffness you have experienced during the last week in your knee. Stiffness is a sensation of restriction or slowness in the ease with which you move your knee joint.

S6. How sever is your knee joint stiffness after first wakening in the morning?

None ☐   Mild ☐   Moderate ☐   Severe ☐   Extreme ☐

Figure 8.7 A more complex questionnaire: the KOOS knee survey.

Reprinted from E.M. Roos and L.S. Lohmander, 2012, *Knee injury and osteoarthritis outcome score (KOOS)*.

S7. How severe is your knee stiffness after sitting, lying or resting later in the day?

None ☐ Mild ☐ Moderate ☐ Severe ☐ Extreme ☐

Pain

P1. How often do you experience knee pain?

Never ☐ Monthly ☐ Weekly ☐ Daily ☐ Always ☐

What amount of knee pain have you experienced the last week during the following activities?

P2. Twisting/pivoting on your knee

None ☐ Mild ☐ Moderate ☐ Severe ☐ Extreme ☐

P3. Straightening knee fully

None ☐ Mild ☐ Moderate ☐ Severe ☐ Extreme ☐

P4. Bending knee fully

None ☐ Mild ☐ Moderate ☐ Severe ☐ Extreme ☐

P5. Walking on flat surface

None ☐ Mild ☐ Moderate ☐ Severe ☐ Extreme ☐

P6. Going up or down stairs.

None ☐ Mild ☐ Moderate ☐ Severe ☐ Extreme ☐

P7. At night while in bed

None ☐ Mild ☐ Moderate ☐ Severe ☐ Extreme ☐

P8. Sitting or lying

None ☐ Mild ☐ Moderate ☐ Severe ☐ Extreme ☐

P9. Standing upright

None ☐ Mild ☐ Moderate ☐ Severe ☐ Extreme ☐

Function, daily living

The following questions concern your physical function. By this we mean your ability to move around and to look after yourself. For each of the following activities please indicate the degree of difficulty you have experienced in the last week due to your knee.

A1. Descending stairs

None ☐ Mild ☐ Moderate ☐ Severe ☐ Extreme ☐

Figure 8.7 *(continued)*

KOOS Knee Survey *(continued)*

A2 Ascending stairs

None ☐ Mild ☐ Moderate ☐ Severe ☐ Extreme ☐

For each of the following activities please indicate the degree of difficulty you have experienced in the last week due to your knee.

A3. Rising from sitting

None ☐ Mild ☐ Moderate ☐ Severe ☐ Extreme ☐

A4. Standing

None ☐ Mild ☐ Moderate ☐ Severe ☐ Extreme ☐

A5. Bending to floor/pick up an object

None ☐ Mild ☐ Moderate ☐ Severe ☐ Extreme ☐

A6. Walking on flat surface

None ☐ Mild ☐ Moderate ☐ Severe ☐ Extreme ☐

A7. Getting in/out of car

None ☐ Mild ☐ Moderate ☐ Severe ☐ Extreme ☐

A8. Going shopping

None ☐ Mild ☐ Moderate ☐ Severe ☐ Extreme ☐

A9. Putting on socks/stockings

None ☐ Mild ☐ Moderate ☐ Severe ☐ Extreme ☐

A10. Rising from bed

None ☐ Mild ☐ Moderate ☐ Severe ☐ Extreme ☐

A11. Taking off socks/stockings

None ☐ Mild ☐ Moderate ☐ Severe ☐ Extreme ☐

A12. Lying in bed (turning over, maintaining knee position)

None ☐ Mild ☐ Moderate ☐ Severe ☐ Extreme ☐

A13. Getting in/out of bath

None ☐ Mild ☐ Moderate ☐ Severe ☐ Extreme ☐

A14. Sitting

None ☐ Mild ☐ Moderate ☐ Severe ☐ Extreme ☐

A15. Getting on/off toilet

None ☐ Mild ☐ Moderate ☐ Severe ☐ Extreme ☐

Figure 8.7 *(continued)*

For each of the following activities please indicate the degree of difficulty you have experienced in the last week due to your knee.

A16. Heavy domestic duties (moving heavy boxes, scrubbing floors, etc.)

None ☐   Mild ☐   Moderate ☐   Severe ☐   Extreme ☐

A17. Light domestic duties (cooking, dusting, etc.)

None ☐   Mild ☐   Moderate ☐   Severe ☐   Extreme ☐

Function, sports and recreational activities

The following questions concern your physical function when being active on a higher level. The questions should be answered thinking of what degree of difficulty you have experienced during the last week due to your knee.

SP1. Squatting

None ☐   Mild ☐   Moderate ☐   Severe ☐   Extreme ☐

SP2. Running

None ☐   Mild ☐   Moderate ☐   Severe ☐   Extreme ☐

SP3. Jumping

None ☐   Mild ☐   Moderate ☐   Severe ☐   Extreme ☐

SP4. Twisting/pivoting on your injured knee

None ☐   Mild ☐   Moderate ☐   Severe ☐   Extreme ☐

SP5. Kneeling

None ☐   Mild ☐   Moderate ☐   Severe ☐   Extreme ☐

Quality of Life

Q1. How often are you aware of your knee problem?

Never ☐   Monthly ☐   Weekly ☐   Daily ☐   Constantly ☐

Q2. Have you modified your life style to avoid potentially damaging activities to your knee?

Not at all ☐   Mildly ☐   Moderately ☐   Severely ☐   Totally ☐

Q3. How much are you troubled with lack of confidence in your knee?

Not at all ☐   Mildly ☐   Moderately ☐   Severely ☐   Extremely ☐

Q4. In general, how much difficulty do you have with your knee?

None ☐   Mild ☐   Moderate ☐   Severe ☐   Extreme

Figure 8.7   *(continued)*

Outcome Score (KOOS), which is available free of charge and assesses symptoms, stiffness, pain, daily living function, sport and recreational activity function, and quality of life.[14] This instrument gives a subcategory score for each section and an overall score, given the same 5-point Likert scale for each question in the instrument.

Athletic trainers are currently working to demonstrate the value of their services to gain point-of-care reimbursement privileges. By consistently using of one or more of these outcome measures that assess change in an injured athlete's condition, from the athlete's point of view, we can easily demonstrate and quantify the value of athletic training services. Thus, once you find a psychometrically sound outcome instrument that suits your practice, use it regularly and keep records of the outcome data for future use with administrative efforts to improve workplace situations.

Adjusting Your Practice

If you have put forth the effort and time to update your clinical practice to include evidence-based practice, this should translate into a culture of lifelong learning that motivates you into EBP action mode every time a clinical question arises. Remember that it will take practice, as with all new skill sets, to become efficient and effective with the EBP skills. When you hit the point of feeling competent and confident with your EBP skills, adjusting your clinical practice should be a regular occurrence. Understanding and using clinical outcome measures will allow you to assess your own outcomes to continually improve your practice.

Setting Time Aside for EBP Searches

The most difficult part of transforming into an EBP clinician is making the time to search for the evidence you need.[10] To this end, it is critical that you write search time into your weekly schedule, if not your daily schedule. If you wait until you have some free time, you will likely find that other tasks fill that time. Thus, just as you set time aside in your daily schedule to review each athlete's progress before each appointment, you could set aside 30 minutes daily to dive into the literature and become better informed about clinical issues you are working on with the athletes in your care. This time needs to be a permanent addition to your schedule if you intend to remain an evidence-based clinician.

Communicating the Latest Research to Your Athletes and Staff

If your athletes do not value the care you provide, you should not be providing that care. To learn how your care is valued, you need to engage in communication—both listening and sharing—with your athletes to let them know that you value their assessment. This occurs when you ask injured athletes how they are doing when they arrive daily. It occurs when you give them choices regarding their exercises that day. And it occurs when you let them know that you care enough about them to search the literature for the latest evidence regarding the treatment of their condition.

Additionally, sharing important evidence that you've discovered with colleagues can improve athletic training services for others besides just those under your care. Perhaps you find new evidence regarding treatment for patellar tendinosis and share that with other basketball athletic trainers in your collegiate conference. Perhaps you find evidence regarding a new and improved clinical diagnostic test for growth plate fractures in young athletes, which you share with all of the high school athletic trainers in your school district or state. Or perhaps you perform an extensive EBP search on treatment methods for medial elbow epicondylitis and decide to create a critically appraised topic (CAT) report to share with your baseball athletic trainer colleagues. Whatever the case, if you find any type of evidence that is important to you and may change your practice, there is a strong likelihood that it will also be important to other athletic trainers. Communicating new findings to your athletes and colleagues will serve your athletic training community well into the future.

Keeping Apprised of the Latest Research Evidence

As we've stated many times throughout this text, the amount of research being produced in any given field is staggering and presents an insurmountable amount of reading for any clinician. This underscores the utility of systematic reviews, meta-analyses, critically appraised topics, and clinical practice guidelines. Each of these resources should be sought during initial EBP searches. Only after determining that these types of reports are not available should you rely on basic independent research studies, such as randomized controlled trials.

Other tools to keep you apprised of the latest research include RSS feeds, My NCBI within PubMed, podcasts from journals and professional organizations, and critically appraised topic libraries. These push technology tools (except for CATs) are presented in greater detail in chapter 7. If you have not yet explored these options and set up an RSS feed, for example, then you should do that soon. These tools bring the latest research to your desktop without your having to perform EBP searches.

Summary

This chapter presented an overview of research outcome measures, including questionnaires and performance-based outcome measures. The psychometric properties of these outcome measures are reliability, validity, and clinical meaningfulness. These properties were presented at length to help you understand the importance of determining the quality of the outcome measures you find. Search techniques to find these high-quality outcome instruments were presented, as were strategies to help you communicate the outcomes you use to your athletes, your sports medicine team, and beyond. Finally, we discussed the importance of assessing your self-practice and making changes to your practice to keep current. The purpose of this chapter is to ensure that you not only are capable of performing EBP searches to find the latest evidence but also clearly understand the quality and utility of outcome measures so you can implement them in your daily clinical practice.

References

1. Fetters LK, Tilson J. *Evidence based physical therapy.* Philadelphia: Davis; 2012.

2. Haley SM, Fragala-Pinkham MA. Interpreting change scores of tests and measures used in physical therapy. *Phys Ther.* 2006; 86(5): 735-743.

3. Chapman J, Norvell D, Hermsmeyer J, et al. Evaluating common outcomes for measuring treatment success for chronic low back pain. *Spine.* 2011; 36 (21 suppl): 54-66.

4. Gliner J, Morgan G. *Research methods in applied settings: An integrated approach to design and analysis.* Mahwah, NJ: Lawrence Erlbaum; 2000.

5. van den Akker-Scheek I, Seldentuis A, Reininga I, Stevens M. Reliability and validity of the Dutch version of the Foot and Ankle Outcome Score (FAOS). *BMC Musculoskelet Disord.* 2013; 14: 183-188.

6. Crosby R, Kolotkin R, Williams G. Defining clinically meaningful change in health-related quality of life. *J Clin Epidemiol.* 2003; 56: 395-407.

7. Jaeschke R, Singer J, Guyatt GA. Measurement of health status: Ascertaining the minimal clinically important difference. *Control Clin Trials.* 1989; 10: 407-409.

8. Kean C, Birmingham T, Garland S, Bryant D, Giffin J. Minimal detectable change in quadriceps strength and voluntary muscle activation in patients with knee osteoarthritis. *Arch Phys Med Rehab.* 2010; 91 (9): 1447-1451.

9. Tashjian R, Deloach J, Green A, Porucznik C, Powell A. Minimal clinically important differences in ASES and simple shoulder test scores after nonoperative treatment of rotator cuff disease. *J Bone Jt Surg Am.* 2010; 92 (2): 296-297.

10. Hankemeier D, Van Lunen B. Perceptions of approved clinical instructors: Barriers in the implementation of evidence-based practice. *J Athl Train.* 2013; 48 (3): 382-393.

11. Welch C, Hankemeier D, Wyant A, Hays D, Pitney W, Van Lunen B. Future directions of evidence-based practice in athletic training: Perceived strategies. *J Athl Train.* 2014; 49 (2): 234-244.

12. Eechaute C, Vaes P, Van Aerschot L, Asman S, Duquet W. The clinimetric qualities of patient-assessed instruments for measuring chronic ankle instability: A systematic review. *BMC Musculoskelet Disord.* 2007; 18 (8): 6-12.

13. Global Rating of Change Scale (GROC). Cisco LifeConnections Health Center website. www.cisco.com/web/lchc/assets/pdf/GROC.pdf. Updated 2014. Accessed May 28, 2014.

14. Roos EM, Lohmander LS. Knee Injury and Osteoarthritis Outcome Score (KOOS). Knee Injury and Osteoarthritis Outcome Score website. www.koos.nu. Published 2012. Updated 2012. Accessed May 28, 2014.

PART III

Research Statistics and Design

The chapters in part III were written for those who want—or are required—to pursue a greater understanding of basic research statistics and design in athletic training. Understanding designs and the types of statistics used in those designs is very helpful when reading and appraising research studies. This section does not include all the information necessary for performing high-quality research. Rather, it is intended to help you become a good consumer of research. Part III will further help you critically appraise the evidence you find and are considering implementing in your clinical practice.

Chapter 9 provides a concise description of quantitative research designs and methods and associated common statistical measures. Entire textbooks have been written on this topic, but we have attempted to condense and present only the most critical aspects. Examples in athletic training research are presented to increase your understanding of specific topics. A critical appraisal is offered to demonstrate how to evaluate quantitative research studies.

Chapter 10 provides a concise description of qualitative research designs and methods, as well as data analysis. Chapter 9 describes quantitative research, which uses numbers to evaluate a topic, whereas chapter 10 describes qualitative research, which uses words to describe meaning within a topic. Both types of research have a place in athletic training, depending on the topic to be studied. Chapter 10 ends with a critical appraisal example to demonstrate how to evaluate qualitative research studies.

Finally, chapter 11 reviews research ethics, including a brief history of the evolution of ethical research practices, followed by an explanation of how those historical lessons continue to inform our research today. Scenarios are presented to demonstrate both sound and questionable research practices.

A discussion of the purpose and function of institutional review boards concludes the chapter.

Part III adds the last few concepts necessary for a complete understanding of basics in evidence-based practice in the profession of athletic training.

CHAPTER 9

Quantitative Research

Objectives

After reading this chapter, you will be able to do the following:

- Describe the types of quantitative data.
- Describe the types of quantitative research designs.
- Explain the purpose of a sampling plan.
- Understand the commonly reported descriptive statistics.
- Interpret common inferential statistics.

Researchers commonly prefer one type of research, either quantitative or qualitative. The depth of skill required to conduct either effectively may serve as a limit to many researchers preferring one to the other. Both types have their advantages, and the choice of which to use is best determined by the goals of the research or the question to be answered. Neither type should be seen as superior because both can answer important questions related to health care. **Quantitative research** uses numbers and mathematical equations to test hypotheses in an unbiased manner. It involves objective data such as distance, temperature, and scales. Qualitative research, which is discussed in chapter 10, involves rich descriptors and attempts to understand people's behavior and experiences. Unlike quantitative research, qualitative research is not limited to items that can be objectively measured while remaining detached from the subject; the qualitative researcher becomes involved with and intimately studies the subjects.

Recently, the medical fields have experienced a push to base clinical decisions on outcomes and empirical evidence. This has challenged seasoned health care providers who continue to use tried-and-true traditional treatments. Some are being required to move away from personal preference and procedures they have found comfortable and used intuitively.[1] Evidence-based practice is requiring health care providers and athletic trainers to conduct quantitative studies to compare the effectiveness of techniques or treatments, both old and new. This chapter explores the steps required to understand and potentially initiate systematic evaluations of interventions used in the athletic training room.

Types of Quantitative Data

As you embark on reading about quantitative research or consider performing your own, remember that you will be assessing an objective measure (e.g., distance, temperature, vital capacity, heart rate). Numbers are not always equal; for example, a 1-unit change in distance is not the same as a 1-unit change in pressure. All measurements can be classified into categories, which will affect later statistical evaluations. The four levels of data are nominal, ordinal, interval, and ratio.[1]

Let's start by reviewing the nominal level of data. As the term *nominal* implies, this is simply a category that provides names to variables. The names lack any significant meaning and do not imply order or quality. Imagine that you want to assess the test performance of two groups. You call one group A and the other group B. This is just for convenience; you could have just as easily called them group X and group XX. Another example is a student project that involves asking students at the university dining facility whether they drink alcohol. The student researcher would end up with a survey response showing the number of yes and no responses. Although she can then place these students into categories of drinkers and nondrinkers, she is missing lots of data about them, such as how often and how much they drink, when they last drank, why they drink, and what types of drinks they prefer.

Foundations of Evidence: Levels of Data

- **Nominal level (weakest level):** The most basic level provides simply a name, not an order or value. For example, a football player with the number 10 on his jersey is not half the person the player with the number 20 is. The number is just an identifier.

- **Ordinal level:** This level uses labels, but they have an order structure (e.g., freshman football = 0, JV football = 1, and varsity football = 2). In this case, the values do not represent skill or ability. A varsity player is not 2 times older, faster, or more skilled than a JV player with the assigned number of 1. The numbers represent an order and not a set distance.

- **Interval level:** A preferred measurement that presents the information of the nominal and ordinal scales but has consistent values (e.g., the difference between 5 feet and 10 feet is the same as the distance between 20 feet and 25 feet).

- **Ratio level:** The optimum measure that presents all previous data discussed in nominal, ordinal, and interval levels but offers additional data. Ratios contain zeros, which can be meaningful. Consider two reductions in swelling of 0 cm and 2 cm. The latter can be stated as a ratio or fraction; it was twice the reduction of the former.

Based on Hicks 2009.

The **ordinal** level of data tells us a little bit more than the nominal level does. An example of ordinal data is the results of a questionnaire using a Likert ranking scale. Using the alcohol example, the student researcher might now ask, How many alcoholic drinks do you consume in a week? The answer choices are *Fewer than 3 (seldom), Fewer than 6 (moderate), Fewer than 9 (heavy),* and *More than 9 (excessive).* These categories are ranked; that is, they can be placed in ascending order. Student grades are another example of ordinal data. It is understood that a student who has earned an A has performed better than a student who has earned a B or a C. These letters have ranks, although they don't represent exact measures. The A student might have performed at 100% and the B student at 80%; or the A student might have performed at 90% and the B student at 89%. In this example you can see that ordinal data reveal rank but not how far apart in rank the items are. Another example of ordinal data in survey research is the age of participants. Researchers often ask respondents to select their age based on a scale—for example, 18 to 28 years, 29 to 38 years, 39 to 48 years, 49 to 58 years, 59 and older. This provides the number of respondents in the age categories but not their actual ages. Therefore, this data can't be averaged or computed.

Moving up the levels of data, we come to the **interval** level. The nice thing about interval data is that the distance between the variables is the same. Reviewing our grade example, because we did not know whether the A student had performed at 90% or 100% or whether the B student had performed at 80% or 89%, we could not compute the difference between them. On an interval scale, we would know the students' exact grades and could calculate how many percentage points separated them. A zero on an interval scale doesn't mean the total absence of what is being measured. Let's look at a pain scale. If a researcher is measuring the change in pain on a scale of 0 to 10 and an athlete reports pain at level 1 today and at level 1 tomorrow, he has a change of zero points. This does not mean he has zero pain.

The highest level of data is ratio data. **Ratio** data has all the qualities of the previous levels of data but also has a true zero. It includes measures such as distance, weight, and time. If you have traveled zero meters, you are referring to an absolute zero, unlike the zero in the example about pain. However, for the sake of statistics and calculations, interval and ratio data are treated the same.

When reviewing an article or collecting your own data, collect as much data in as much detail as possible. Also, try to collect interval or ratio data and not nominal or ordinal data. If you ask participants to rate themselves as young, middle aged, or old, you cannot later extrapolate their actual ages and use these values parametrically to calculate means. However, if you collect participants' ages so that you have a continuum between 1 and the age of the oldest person completing your study, you have interval data. At a later time you could collapse those ages into the categories of young (below 30), middle aged (31-50), and old (50 and older).

Parametric and Nonparametric Data

The four types of data are further categorized as parametric or nonparametric. Interval and ratio data are parametric. **Parametric** means that the values fall in a normal distribution, allowing researchers to draw conclusions mathematically. A normal distribution is symmetrical around its mean. If we took the temperature of

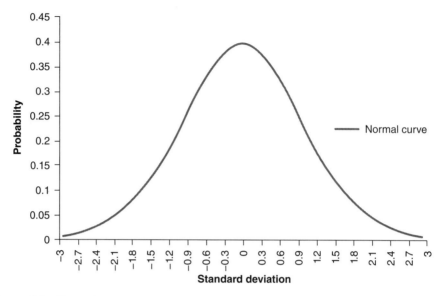

Figure 9.1 Normal curve.

100 people, we would expect the mean temperature to be 98.6. Figure 9.1 shows a normal curve that extends on the x-axis from –3 to 0 and then to 3. Approximately 68% of all of people's temperatures would fall from –1 to 1 on the x-axis. This is referred to as a standard deviation (SD) of 1. As we move out to an SD of –2 and 2, we would capture 95.4 % of our values; at SD 3 and –3, we would capture 95.6% of our values. Let's assume that an SD of 1 would capture temperatures between 97.6 and 99.6, and an SD of 2 would capture temperatures between 96.6 and 100.6. This would account for approximately 95% of our sample of 100 people. This tells you that the extreme temperatures of, say, 95.6 or 101.6 are less likely to occur and are not likely in a normal sample.

When researchers look at the results of an intervention, they collect baseline data, or controls, which are often normally distributed values. After a treatment or intervention, they want to see new values that fall to one extreme or another near an SD of 3. This means that there is approximately a 95% chance that this finding is rare or that the treatment actually had an impact on the measurement of interest.

Nominal and ordinal categories of data are considered **nonparametric** because they are not normally distributed. Histograms, bar graphs, and pie charts are often used to present nonparametric values.

Measures of Central Tendency

To fully understand quantitative analysis and normal curve distributions, you need to understand **measures of central tendency**. The measures of central tendency revolve around the mean, median, and mode, and these values cluster around the center of the normal distribution. Reviewing our previous example of temperature and figure 9.1, you'll notice that 68% of all the scores revolve around the center. In a normal distribution, this is where you will find the mean, median, and mode. The **arithmetic mean** is the average of all scores and is normally denoted in articles by the symbol $\overline{x}$.[1] Keep in mind that the mean can be skewed by scores that fall on either side of a normal distribution.

Referencing the 100 people whose temperatures we took, let's say that one person was being treated for hypothermia and had a temperature of 91 °F (32.8 °C). This would be a rare occurrence, but in this sample it would decrease the mean. In a class of 50 people taking a test, the mean score might be 70. This would look poor if the goal was to average 90%, but if one or two people scored 0% and the rest of the class scored 90% or better, those two zeros would skew the mean. For this reason, it is often prudent to look at the **median score**, or the score that falls in the middle of the distribution. Using the test score example, if 48 people scored 90% and 2 scored 0%, your median score, or the 25th score (the one in the middle of the distribution), would be 90%. The **mode** is the most commonly occurring value in a distribution of numeric data. It helps researchers answer certain types of questions. For example, if a researcher wanted to know the age of college students experiencing an ACL injury, the mode, or the age that occurred most often, would be the most helpful measure.

Quantitative Research Designs

The quantitative researcher's general goal is to establish the presence of a relationship between measures of interest. Quantitative research studies usually involve **independent variables** (IVs) and **dependent variables** (DVs). Independent variables don't change (e.g., a person's race or level of education). A DV can change based on the outcome of the intervention or treatment; for this reason, it is often the measure of interest. To avoid variability and to be able to make comparisons and draw conclusions, researchers must control the study environment other than the variable being studied. Quantitative research is often used to measure statistically significant differences in groups over time. The key is that most variables are controlled; only the one being evaluated is allowed to change. This enables the researcher to say that a certain intervention caused the change. Quantitative research designs fall into the categories of descriptive, quasi-experimental, and experimental.[2] Deciding which is appropriate depends on the research question.

Descriptive research involves correlational and evaluative data assessment. These both involve collecting data that are typically numeric to answer a question or describe the current status of the participants. Evaluative questions might be What do athletic trainers think about rectal temperature assessment in middle and high school–aged athletes? or Why do athletic trainers continue to tape ankles when most research studies show that tape loses its function in 10 to 15 minutes? Correlational questions might be What is the relationship between strength and injury rates? or What is the relationship between flexibility and muscle tears? With evaluative questions, it is important to remember that the researcher doesn't start with a hypothesis. The same is true of correlational questions, which simply present correlations. It would be inappropriate to say that one variable causes the other.

Quasi-experimental studies attempt to establish a cause-and-effect relationship between variables. The differences between quasi- and true experimental designs are that quasi-designs lack random assignment and the IV is not manipulated to change the DV. The researcher wants to know whether the naturally occurring IV has a significant effect on the DV. Questions answered by quasi-experimental designs are similar to those answered by correlational designs, but instead of a relationship, the researcher is looking for an effect. A correlational question might be What is the relationship between flexibility and injury rates? As a quasi-experimental question, it would be What effect does flexibility have on injury rates? The weakness here is that nothing else is controlled for (e.g., participants' age, sex, weight, or strength). That means that even if flexibility appears to affect injury rates, the researcher could not be certain because other variables were not controlled.

The final category of quantitative design is **true experimental**. True experimental studies control for all the other variables of interest, allowing the researcher to seek evidence about a particular intervention or treatment. They are often thought to be the gold standard of research methods.[2] To change the study of flexibility and injury rate to an experimental design, you would need to recruit participants of the same age, same sex, and same level of sport participation with no current injuries. Then you would assess their flexibility and randomly assign half to a control group not doing stretching exercises and half to an intervention group performing stretching exercises. Everything else about their training program remains the same, and you follow them for a season or two. At the end of that time, you look at the number of injuries in the two groups to see whether the stretching program had an impact on injury rates.

Even the best of research designs will leave researchers with meaningless studies if they fail to consider generalizability, which is influenced by sample size and population representation. **Generalizability** pertains to reliability by asking whether the reported measure or outcome can be reproduced. When appraising research, you want to know whether the results are reproducible and, more important, whether you can reproduce them with your athlete. Let's assume that a technique to graft damaged skin worked in a population of healthy children between the ages of 8 and 12 who were burned by fire. You might assume that the technique could apply to boys of the same age group who suffer skin damage from sliding into a base while playing baseball. However, if you are dealing with a geriatric athlete who also has diabetes, the technique might not be effective because the study is not generalizable to your population.

Researchers should inform their readers of the demographics of their study participants to help them make generalizability decisions. They should report the sample size and whether it was representative of the population of interest. The National Athletic Trainers' Association (NATA) has more than 30,000 members. If a researcher wants to know how members feel about the NATA president, asking every NATA member would not be feasible. To avoid a timely and costly attempt at polling an entire population, researchers determine a **representative sample**, which is a subset of the entire population that would reflect that population. A sampling plan can be approached in many ways. An important consideration is whether the sample is large enough to ensure that it reflects all the ideas or items of interest in a population.[1] In the NATA example, if you ask only 10 people, you might, by chance alone, get similar thoughts and miss what a majority of members think. Another important consideration in sampling is reaching an entire demographic of the population. Let's say that a researcher asks 300 NATA members what they think of the president, but all of these participants reside in Michigan, the home state of the NATA president. These results might not reflect what members in California or Arizona think.

To address these sampling issues and ensure a representative sample, researchers develop sampling plans before collecting any data. Researchers might use incidental sampling, stratified sampling, or systemic sampling.[1]

Incidental sampling is also referred to as convenience sampling because it involves sampling from a population you have access to.[1] This may not be truly random across an entire population, which may affect the results, but it is commonly used for logistical reasons. Consider a researcher at a university who wants to know if a new therapy treatment will help resolve the issues associated with chronic ankle instability. She decides to sample from the athletes at her institution. This is very convenient but might not represent all the athletes playing at the college level across the country.

Stratified sampling requires the researcher to know the proportions of subgroups within a population. Using the NATA data, let's assume that the NATA membership is 33,000 and the researcher needs 10% of the population to participate in a survey. This means that the researcher needs 3,300 members to complete the survey. A simple approach would be to randomly survey 3,300 NATA members. The problem is that districts have substantially different member populations. Using stratified sampling, you would need to know the percentage of 33,000 who belong to each of the 10 districts. If district 9 makes up 27% of the NATA membership, 27% of 33,000 is 8,910 members. Ten percent of 8,910 is 891. By surveying members in each district in this way, you ensure that you get 10% from each and that no district has a greater representation.

Systemic sampling is not entirely random, but it can produce a representative sample. It involves establishing an interval and sampling every person in a population who falls along that interval. A researcher who wants to survey 10% of the NATA membership may survey every 10th person across the entire set of 33,000. This would result in a survey of 3,300 members, or 10%.

Descriptive Statistics

Descriptive statistics provide a simple but powerful way to describe your data to readers. Descriptive statistics allow you to condense large amounts of data about a population and present them in an organized fashion. A few common methods are tables, graphs, bar graphs, and pie charts. Tables are helpful for presenting large amounts of data in a way that is easy to interpret. In table 9.1 you can quickly and clearly see that soccer players had the most ACL injuries between 2009 and 2013, and that 2011 was the year of the most injuries across the sports.

A line chart is a simple graph that allows readers to quickly assess rates. Figure 9.2 shows what appears to be a trend of increasing elbow surgeries. A bar graph is

Table 9.1　ACL Injuries per Sport for Five Years

	2009	2010	2011	2012	2013	Total
Football	4	3	5	1	2	15
Soccer	3	4	5	3	4	19
Basketball	0	2	1	0	1	4
Total	7	9	11	4	7	

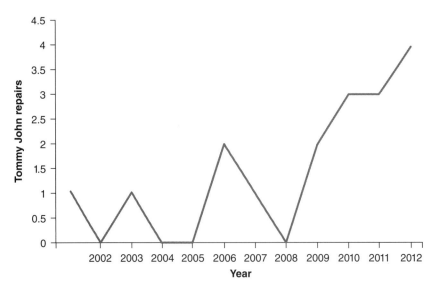

Figure 9.2 Line chart.

another graph that allows readers to visualize data. Figure 9.3 may be a bar graph that an athletic director created to show coaches the number of athletes in each grade at a high school or college. Showing percentages is easily accomplished with a pie chart. Readers can see the percentages of people in a whole sample or population who fall into certain categories. Figure 9.4 reveals that people with MA degrees make up the largest percentage of NATA members (71%).

Common Inferential Statistics

Although a plethora of statistical methods exists in the literature, a few of the most common are discussed here to help you understand what's being reported. The methods addressed in this section are correlations, t-tests, ANOVA, and regression.

Correlations

Correlations, as discussed in chapter 3, simply show a relationship and are reported as *r*; absolute values closer to 1 show higher correlations. The meaningfulness, or clinical appropriateness, of the relationship depends on the study and what is being assessed. When reviewing parametric statistics, remember that they all assume that the data are normally distributed.[3]

t-Tests

An independent t-test is used to compare a single measure on two levels (before and after treatment). Let's assume that a researcher is interested in the pain reported by 60 athletes who have sustained a second-degree ankle sprain. The single measure of interest is pain, and the two levels are those being treated and those not being treated. At baseline the researcher splits the group randomly into two groups of

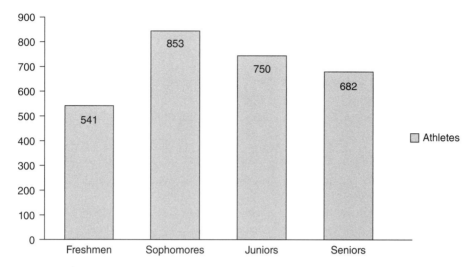

Figure 9.3 Bar graph.

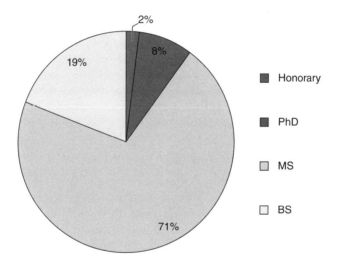

Figure 9.4 Pie chart.

30. One group is treated with ice, and the other is not. After the ice treatments, the athletes report their pain score. The researcher suspects that if the ice diminished pain, the average pain score of the group being treated with ice would be lower than that of the group not being treated. If the calculation of the t-test shows no significant difference in the pain scores, the researcher would conclude that the ice treatments failed to reduce pain. However, if the difference in the values between the groups is significant, and the mean pain score of those being iced was lower, the researcher would report that ice did significantly reduce pain in this particular sample.

The t-test is limited to simple, one-dimensional comparisons. Moreover, only one t-test should be performed on a set of data. Consider a researcher who has collected participant data on age (over or under 30), injury history (yes or no), education level (high school or college), sport participation (yes or no), and handedness (left or right). The researcher wants to look at each of these and see if there is a difference in sex (e.g., do males have more injuries than females, or do females have a higher education average than males). This would be simple to calculate but is likely to result in a family-wise error.

Chapter 5 discussed p values and how to determine whether a significant finding occurred by chance alone (i.e., was not the result of a true difference). During a t-test calculation, the researcher finds a p value; a value greater than .05 is typically interpreted as nonsignificant because the difference between the means might be just from chance. If the p value is less than .05 or .01, the difference in the scores is less likely to have occurred by chance alone, and the difference in the means is interpreted as significant.

Let's look at p values in a practical sense. The p value tells you the likelihood of getting the same result at least 95 times if you repeated the study 100 times. With that in mind, think about a bucket with 100 marbles in it—95 white ones and 5 red ones. Your task is to pull out one marble. Pulling out a white marble means that you made a good decision or interpretation; a red marble means that you made an error. When you pull out the first marble, you have a 95% chance of grabbing a white marble, or making a correct interpretation. There are now 99 marbles in the bucket (94 white and 5 red), so the next time you pull one out, you have a higher chance of grabbing a red one. In the same way, every time you run a comparison using a t-test in the example of values between male and female, you run a higher chance of creating an error. Therefore, anytime you are assessing an article that reports the use of multiple t-tests, make sure that they have been performed on independent sets of data or that the author presents a mathematical correction to account for and acknowledge the chance of creating an error.

ANOVA

An analysis of variance (ANOVA) is more versatile than a t-test because it allows you to compare more than one set of means at a time and decrease the fear of committing a family-wise error. When using a t-test, the researcher has one DV and one IV, and the DV is treated as continuous. When using an ANOVA, the researcher can have more than two IVs. This allows for comparisons beyond a dichotomous situation such as ice or no ice. A two-way ANOVA is the same except that you can have two or more IVs, each of which can have two or more levels. ANOVAs also generate p values that are interpreted the same way as described in chapter 5 or as t-tests. A MANOVA is a statistical test beyond the scope of this text. Suffice it to say that it allows researchers to compare studies with more than one DV and variable numbers of IVs.

Regression

The final common inferential statistic is regression. Regression is useful when a researcher knows the relationships among numerous variables and wants to predict the values of another.[1] Regression can be very useful for those researching common concerns in athletic training.

Let's assume that an athletic trainer at a college knows the age, quadriceps and hamstring strength ratios, Q angle, lower-extremity flexibility, and rate of lower-extremity injuries of over 500 soccer players. He can compare these to each other using a correlation, but doing so will not reveal a cause and effect if one exists. The real questions are Do any of these variables influence the rate of lower-extremity injuries? and Could we prophylactically change any of these variables and decrease the rate of injury? Regression is the perfect tool for answering these questions. The athletic trainer enters the values for all the IVs and then determines the DV of lower-extremity injury rate. He then calculates mathematically which IV varied the most in alignment with the DV. Although some may have had an impact, regression reveals which variables had the greatest influence on the DV.

With this information in hand, the athletic trainer may do two things. First, he may try to address the issues causing lower-extremity injury. If the predictors are strength and flexibility, then he can address them in a training program to try to decrease injury rates. His other option is predictive. If, during baseline assessments as part of physicals or other events, he discovers athletes with indicators that predispose them to injury, he can develop a plan to decrease or mitigate that risk.

Statistical Power

All of the previously discussed statistical methods rely on statistical power and appropriate sample sizes. In chapter 3, we discussed false negatives and false positives. In figure 9.5, the false positive would be in box B and the false negative in box C.

In this figure, a false positive is the detection of a disease when one is not present, and a false negative is when a disease does exist but is not detected. Both box B and box C represent assessment errors. When assessing power, we want to determine whether to reject or accept our hypothesis. Using the example of using ice and decreasing pain, let's assume that our hypothesis is that ice decreases pain. In this instance, we want to find support that this hypothesis (H) is true (figure 9.6).

Remember that false negatives and false positives are errors. The same is true here when assessing our power to accept or reject our hypothesis. If we reject a true hypothesis, we have committed a type I error (i.e., ice does decrease pain, but we failed to have enough subjects in our study to detect that difference). Our false

		DISEASE	
		+	−
NEW TEST	+	A (True positive)	B (False positive)
	−	C (False negative)	D (True negative)

Figure 9.5 New test and disease 2× 2 table.

	REAL TRUTH	
	H is true	H is false
ACCEPT H	OK	Type II error probability β
REJECT H	Type I error probability α	OK

Figure 9.6 Real truth 2× 2 table.

conclusion would be that ice does not decrease pain. If we accept a hypothesis that in real life is not true, we have committed a type II error (i.e., ice does not reduce pain, but as a result of our sample size, we determined that it does). The probability of committing these errors is calculated using β (beta) and α (alpha). These are inversely related—as alpha, or your risk of committing a type I error, goes up, your risk of committing a type II error goes down, and vice versa. The estimation and calculation of power are beyond the scope of this textbook; for a more detailed discussion, see *Research Methods in Physical Activity*.[4]

Your power determines your required sample size, or the number of subjects you need to correctly accept your hypothesis. For an easy example, let's assume that an **a priori** power analysis says that you will need 200 subjects to complete your study, because a brief literature review reveals that only about 25% of subjects recruited complete a study. Simple math then tells you to recruit 800 subjects so that you will have the 200 needed to complete the study and provide the appropriate power. As referenced earlier, this can be accomplished using your sampling plan and methods.

Foundations of Evidence: Research Design Notation

You will find that knowing research design notation will help you assess the groupings and number of assessments or observations required in a study. The following tables on research design notation are an easy-to-use reference.

Describing Experimental Notation

Symbol	Activity Occurring
R	Random assignment to a group
T	Administering a treatment or intervention
O	Observation or assessment of a variable

Quasi-Experimental Design Notation

Design	Notation	Common statistical analyses
Time series design	$O_1 O_2 O_3 O_4 T O_5 O_6 O_7 O_8$	ANOVA (repeated measure)
Reversal design	$O_1 O_2 T_1 O_3 O_4 T_2 O_5 O_6$	(time series analysis)

Pre-Experimental Design Notation

Design	Notation	Common statistic
One-shot study (two groups)	$T O$	t-test (one sample t-test)
One-group pretest–posttest design	$O_1 T O_2$	t-test (paired t-test)
Static group comparison	$T O_1$ ------ O_2	t-test (two sample independent t-test)

Experimental Design Notation

Design	Notation	Common statistic
Groups design	$R T O_1$ $R O_2$	t-test (two sample independent t-test)
Pretest–posttest groups	$R O_1 T O_2$ $R O_3 O_4$	ANOVA
Pretest-posttest groups	$R O_1 T O_2$ $R O_3 O_4$ $R T O_5$ $R O_6$	ANOVA

Data from Ingersoll C. *Research in athletic training.* Thorofare, NJ: Slack; 2001.

Critical Appraisal of Evidence: Time Series

A **time series** is a collection of quantitative observations that are evenly spaced in time and measured successively. Examples of time series are the continuous monitoring of a person's heart rate, breathing rate, or body temperature or hourly readings of air temperature. Time series analysis is generally used when there are 50 or more data points in a series. These are the goals of time series analysis:

- Description: Identify patterns in correlated data.
- Explanation: Understand and model or diagram the data.
- Forecast: Predict short-term trends from previous patterns (i.e., heart rate increase during sprints or body temperature increase with air temperature increase).

(continued)

Critical Appraisal of Evidence (continued)

- Intervention analysis: Learn how a single event changes the time series.
- Quality control: Determine whether deviations of a specified size indicate a problem (i.e., whether an increase of so many degrees in body temperature can predict heat exhaustion).

Time series are analyzed to understand the underlying structure and function that produce the observations. Understanding the mechanisms of a time series allows a mathematical model to be developed that explains the data in such a way that prediction, monitoring, or control can occur. Learning how to statistically analyze a time series is beyond the scope of this text. However, you can do a simple visual inspection by plotting the observed values against time. This may reveal quantitative aspects.

Summary

Quantitative research uses data driven by numbers to support or fail to support hypotheses or answer questions. Appraising an article to determine whether its results can be used to make clinical decisions requires an understanding of a few important issues. The first is the sampling of participants in the study. Did the author sample randomly? Was the sample large enough to capture the occurrences in the population? Is the sample representative and applicable to your clinical situation? The second issue to understand is the descriptive statistics. Are they clearly presented, and do they paint a picture of the qualities of the participants? Finally, you need to understand the inferential statistics explained. Does the author clearly explain the IVs and DVs and the number or level of each? Are the values reported and determined to be significant or nonsignificant? If the answer to any of these questions is no, the study may not be appropriate to use in your clinical practice.

References

1. Hicks C. *Research methods for clinical therapists, applied project design and analysis.* 5th ed. Churchill Livingstone; 2009.

2. Rubin A, Bellamy J. *Practitioner's guide to using research for evidence-based practice.* 2nd ed. Hoboken, NJ: Wiley; 2012.

3. Gliner J, Morgan G. *Research methods in applied settings: An integrated approach to design and analysis.* Mahwah, New Jersey: Lawrence Erlbaum Assoc., Publ; 2000:465. Accessed May 16, 2014.

4. Thomas, JR, Nelson J, Silverman S. *Research methods in physical activity.* 7th ed. Champaign, IL: Human Kinetics; 2015.

Qualitative Studies

There is much debate within the research community over which study approach is better—quantitative or qualitative. Most researchers lean toward one or the other in their own work. As a consumer of research, however, you need to understand both approaches. Each is valuable with certain clinical questions. As you learned in chapter 9, quantitative research generally uses numbers for data to determine cause and effect in the context of a research question. **Qualitative research**, however, generally uses words as data to determine meaning in the context of a research question.

If we wanted to determine whether more athletes sprained an ankle during practices than during games, we would use a quantitative approach, because counting the incidents of ankle sprain (i.e., numbers) would answer the clinical question. On the other hand, if we wanted to understand what drives athletes to develop eating disorders, numbers would hardly illuminate any aspect of the clinical question. Rather, interviewing athletes who have dealt with eating disorders would provide data in the form of words to answer the clinical question.

There is a place for both types of research approaches in the field of athletic training. This chapter explores the types of qualitative research and how this research is conducted, analyzed, and evaluated to help inform your clinical practice.

Types of Qualitative Research Studies

Performing qualitative research is entirely different from performing quantitative research. To understand those differences, you first need to understand the types of qualitative research. The five types outlined in the following sections provide a deeper understanding of the events or conditions that a person, a group, or an entire culture has experienced. The five types of qualitative studies are ethnographic, grounded theory, phenomenological, case, and biographical.

Foundations of Evidence: Types of Qualitative Research

- Ethnographic studies
- Grounded theory studies
- Phenomenological studies
- Case studies
- Biographical studies

Ethnographic Studies

Ethnography is the study of an intact cultural or social group via observations and a prolonged period spent in the field. The ethnographer watches, listens, and records the voices of the participants with the intent of generating a cultural portrait.[1] An example in athletic training would be a study of the culture of working in the professional baseball setting as an athletic trainer. This would be difficult to study using a quantitative approach, because the primary objective of the study is to derive meaning from participants' experiences within that culture. The researcher would need to spend extended time observing and interviewing athletic trainers who work in the setting. Figure 10.1 offers an example of an ethnographic study.

Conducting ethnographic studies can be difficult because the researcher needs to be granted approval to observe the culture for a prolonged period—weeks, often months, and at times years. If the culture exists in public areas, this is less of a problem; gaining access to medical areas (e.g., athletic training rooms, hospitals), however, is more challenging.

Grounded Theory Studies

A **grounded theory** study requires the researcher to generate a theory that explains some action, interaction, or process. This is accomplished through interviews conducted during multiple visits to the setting or field. The data reduction process then generates multiple interrelated themes, which are used to create a substantive context-specific theory.[1] Figure 10.2 offers an example of a grounded theory study. An example in athletic training would be a study of why football players may not

J Black Stud. 2010;41(2):281-300.

Are sports overemphasized in the socialization process of African American males? A qualitative analysis of former collegiate athletes' perception of sport socialization .

Beamon KK.

⊕ Author information

Abstract

Scholars have noted that an elevated level of sports socialization in the family, neighborhood, and media exists within the African American community, creating an overrepresentation of African American males in certain sports. As a result, African American males may face consequences that are distinctly different from the consequences of those who are not socialized as intensively toward athletics, such as lower levels of academic achievement, higher expectations for professional sports careers as a means to upward mobility, and lower levels of career maturity. This study examines the sport socialization of African American male former collegiate athletes through in-depth ethnographic interviews. The results show that the respondents' perceptions were that their socializing agents and socializing environment emphasized athletics above other roles, other talents, and the development of other skills.

Figure 10.1 Ethnographic study in sports.
Reprinted from PubMed.gov. Available: www.ncbi.nlm.nih.gov/pubmed.

J Athl Train. 2013 Sep-Oct;48(5):668-77. doi: 10.4085/1062-6050-48.3.24.

Fulfillment of work-life balance from the organizational perspective: a case study.

Mazerolle SM[1], Goodman A.

⊕ Author information

Abstract

CONTEXT: Researchers studying work-life balance have examined policy development and implementation to create a family-friendly work environment from an individualistic perspective rather than from a cohort of employees working under the same supervisor.

OBJECTIVE: To investigate what factors influence work-life balance within the National Collegiate Athletic Association (NCAA) Division I clinical setting from the perspective of an athletic training staff.

DESIGN: Qualitative study.

SETTING: Web-based management system.

PATIENTS OR OTHER PARTICIPANTS: Eight athletic trainers (5 men, 3 women; age ≈ 38 ± 7 years) in the NCAA Division I setting. Data Collection and Analysis: Participants responded to a series of questions by journaling their thoughts and experiences. We included data-source triangulation, multiple-analyst triangulation, and peer review to establish data credibility. We analyzed the data via a grounded theory approach.

RESULTS: Three themes emerged from the data. Family-oriented and supportive work environment was described as a workplace that fosters and encourages work-life balance through professionally and personally shared goals. Nonwork outlets included activities, such as exercise and personal hobbies, that provide time away from the role of the athletic trainer. Individualistic strategies reflected that although the athletic training staff must work together and support one another, each staff member must have his or her own personal strategies to manage personal and professional responsibilities.

CONCLUSIONS: The foundation for a successful work environment in the NCAA Division I clinical setting potentially can center on the management style of the supervisor, especially one who promotes teamwork among his or her staff members. Although a family-friendly work environment is necessary for work-life balance, each member of the athletic training staff must have personal strategies in place to fully achieve a balance.

Figure 10.2 Grounded theory study in sports.
Reprinted from PubMed.gov. Available: www.ncbi.nlm.nih.gov/pubmed.

report every concussion they experience during practices and games. Although most of us are aware that this occurs frequently, we have not studied exactly why it occurs from the athlete's perspective.

To perform this hypothetical study, we would need to interview several football players who were suspected of not reporting concussions on one or more occasions. The interviews would need to be conducted after their eligibility for playing was done to ensure openness and honesty. Once we have completed, recorded, and transcribed all the interviews, we would analyze the data and group responses into whatever themes emerged from the athletes' words. With the interview responses coded into themes, we could derive a grand theory to explain the action of not reporting concussions from the athlete's perspective.

Phenomenological Studies

Phenomenological studies describe the meaning people ascribe to certain phenomena, topics, or concepts. The researcher attempts to combine individual experiences to determine a central meaning of, or the essence of, the experience.[1] An example in athletic training is an investigation of burnout in the profession. Indeed, many such studies have been conducted over the years, both qualitatively and quantitatively. The quantitative studies that have been performed have focused on the causes of burnout. However, to really understand burnout in the field of athletic training, a phenomenological study would be ideal. Figure 10.3 offers an example of a phenomenological study.

Case Studies

Case studies investigate a confined topic with a focus on either an individual case or an issue that is illustrated by a case. This provides in-depth information on a topic using various methods. The researcher attempts to situate the topic or case within a larger context or setting.[2] We are all familiar with case studies of unusual medical injuries or illnesses that occur in our athletic training rooms. Qualitative case studies differ in that they seek to describe the meaning of the topic from the participants' perspective. Figure 10.4 offers an example of a qualitative case study.

An example of a qualitative case study in athletic training would be a study to illuminate how anorexia nervosa may affect athletic performance. To use the specific case to illustrate the larger issue, we would interview an athlete with the condition whose athletic performance has declined. Case studies in the qualitative realm use intimate portraits derived from personal experience to illuminate larger issues.[2]

Biographical Studies

A biography is the study of one person's experiences, as told to the researcher in person or via historical documents.[1] Commonly, multiple interviews along with historical documents are used to gather data for the study. Biographies in the sporting world are commonly of professional athletes and well-known coaches. An example in athletic training would be an in-depth look at one of the first female athletic trainers to enter the profession in the 1950s. Matt Webber's book *Dropping the Bucket and Sponge* is the first substantive text on our great profession of athletic training; it contains hundreds of historical document transcriptions.[3] For those interested in biographical research of athletic trainers, this text is a

J Sports Sci Med. 2012 Mar 1;11(1):39-50. eCollection 2012.

Views of adolescent female youth on physical activity during early adolescence.

Yungblut HE[1], Schinke RJ, McGannon KR.

⊕ Author Information

Abstract

Early adolescence is a time when a transition away from sport and physical activity participation is at its highest level among female youth (Hedstrom & Gould, 2004). This has led to the identification of barriers and facilitators of physical activity participation for adolescent females. Consequently there have been calls to overcome barriers and augment facilitators via the creation of gender-relevant programming. Despite these calls and efforts, a gender disparity remains, and a detailed understanding of how girls experience and interpret physical activity within the context of their lives is still lacking. The current project aimed to gain further insight into the foregoing using tenets of Interpretive Phenomenology to further understand the lived physical activity experiences of females during early adolescence, delineating their barriers to participation and the factors enabling participation. Five themes were identified and made into vignettes to facilitate understanding from adolescent females' perspectives: friends or don't know anyone, good or not good enough, fun or not fun; good feeling or gross; and peer support or peer pressure. The physical activity promotion implications for female youth are discussed within the context of these themes.

KEYWORDS: Physical activity; female; qualitative; youth

Figure 10.3 Phenomenological study in sports.

Reprinted from PubMed.gov. Available: www.ncbi.nlm.nih.gov/pubmed.

J Athl Train. 2008 May-Jun;43(3):284-92. doi: 10.4085/1062-6050-43.3.284.

Questioning skills demonstrated by approved clinical instructors during clinical field experiences.

Barnum MG.

⊕ Author information

Abstract

CONTEXT: The current trend in athletic training clinical education places greater emphasis on the quality of interactions occurring between Approved Clinical Instructors (ACIs) and athletic training students (ATSs). Among other attributes, the ability of ACIs to facilitate and direct quality clinical learning experiences may be influenced by the skill with which the ACI is able to use selected teaching strategies.

OBJECTIVE: To gain insight into ACIs' use of questioning as a specific teaching strategy during the clinical education experiences of undergraduate ATSs.

DESIGN: Qualitative case study design involving initial and stimulated-recall interviews, prolonged field observations, and audio recording of ACI-ATS interactions.

SETTING: The primary athletic training facility at one athletic training education program accredited by the Commission on Accreditation of Athletic Training Education.

PATIENTS OR OTHER PARTICIPANTS: The 8 ACI participants included 3 full-time athletic training education program faculty members and 5 graduate-level assistants. The 24 ATS participants included 1 senior, 17 juniors, and 6 sophomores.

DATA COLLECTION AND ANALYSIS: Transcribed data collected from 8 initial interviews, 23 field observations, 23 audio-recorded ACI-ATS interactions and 54 stimulated-recall interviews were analyzed through microscopic, open, and axial coding, as well as coding for process. The cognition level of questions posed by ACIs was analyzed according to Sellappah and colleagues' Question Classification Framework.

RESULTS: The ACI participants posed 712 questions during the 23 observation periods. Of the total questions, 70.37% were classified as low-level cognitive questions and 17.00% as high-level cognitive questions. The remaining 12.64% were classified as other.

CONCLUSIONS: Although all ACIs used questioning during clinical instruction, 2 distinct questioning patterns were identified: strategic questioning and nonstrategic questioning. The way ACIs sequenced questions (their questioning pattern) appeared to be more important than the number of specific cognitive-level questions posed. Nonstrategic questioning appears to support knowledge and comprehension, whereas strategic questioning appears to support critical thinking.

KEYWORDS: athletic training education; clinical education; critical thinking; pedagogy

Figure 10.4 Qualitative case study in sports.

Reprinted from PubMed.gov. Available: www.ncbi.nlm.nih.gov/pubmed.

Am J Physiol Lung Cell Mol Physiol. 2013 Oct 15;305(8):L523-9. doi: 10.1152/ajplung.00176.2013. Epub 2013 Aug 30.

Joseph Barcroft's studies of high-altitude physiology.

West JB.

⊕ Author information

Abstract

Joseph Barcroft (1872-1947) was an eminent British physiologist who made contributions to many areas. Some of his studies at high altitude and related topics are reviewed here. In a remarkable experiment he spent 6 days in a small sealed room while the oxygen concentration of the air gradually fell, simulating an ascent to an altitude of nearly 5,500 m. The study was prompted by earlier reports by J. S. Haldane that the lung secreted oxygen at high altitude. Barcroft tested this by having blood removed from an exposed radial artery during both rest and exercise. No evidence for oxygen secretion was found, and the combination of 6 days incarceration and the loss of an artery was heroic. To obtain more data, Barcroft organized an expedition to Cerro de Pasco, Peru, altitude 4,300 m, that included investigators from both Cambridge, UK and Harvard. Again oxygen secretion was ruled out. The protocol included neuropsychometric measurements, and Barcroft famously concluded that all dwellers at high altitude are persons of impaired physical and mental powers, an assertion that has been hotly debated. Another colorful experiment in a low-pressure chamber involved reducing the pressure below that at the summit of Mt. Everest but giving the subjects 100% oxygen to breathe while exercising as a climber would on Everest. The conclusion was that it would be possible to reach the summit while breathing 100% oxygen. Barcroft was exceptional for his self-experimentation under hazardous conditions.

KEYWORDS: exercise at altitude; hypoxia; neuropsychometric measurements; oxygen secretion; permanent residents of high altitude

Figure 10.5 Biographical study in sports.

Reprinted from PubMed.gov. Available: www.ncbi.nlm.nih.gov/pubmed.

valuable resource because it includes many brief biographical transcripts of the profession's forefathers. Documents such as Webber's text are commonly used when writing biographical qualitative studies. Figure 10.5 offers an interesting example of a biographical study.

Gathering Data

As we dig deeper into understanding qualitative research, we need to address the issue of data gathering. With quantitative studies, significant efforts are made to avoid researcher bias and ensure random sampling (if possible) and anonymity (at times). In qualitative studies, these issues are approached very differently—which is a cause of tension between qualitative and quantitative researchers.

Purposeful Sampling

Purposeful sampling may be defined as the process by which the qualitative researcher chooses participants based on their exposure to or experience with the research topic.[1] Recall that in quantitative research, random sampling is highly regarded to avoid researcher bias and to be able to generalize the study outcomes. In qualitative studies, however, researchers state their biases up front and purposefully choose participants who will lend meaning to the topic. The study outcomes simply paint a portrait of the topic based on the researchers' findings. Researcher bias is assumed and is normal. Thus, purposeful sampling is essential to create valid qualitative studies. Other types of sampling used in qualitative research, which are typically subsets of purposeful sampling, are beyond the scope of this text.

Interviewing and Observing

Once the participants have been selected and have agreed to take part in the research, one or a combination of techniques is used to gather the data: interview, observation, and historical document review. Interviews are the most common method of data collection.[2,4] The interviews are usually quite lengthy, often several hours at a time. Most researchers record the interviews and then have the recordings transcribed.

The interview questions must be the same for all participants, but they must be open-ended questions to allow for significant differences in responses. For example, a researcher interviewing one of the first female athletic trainers in the profession might say, "Tell me what prompted you to begin a career in athletic training." The response may last an hour or more. And as the person is responding, the researcher may think of some unscripted questions that would provide more insight. This is normal practice during qualitative studies.

The purpose of interviewing is to get the fullest picture possible from a participant about the topic. This picture will be quite different from those provided by other participants; those differences are essential to qualitative methodology. Getting a full, rich picture of the grander topic from these multiple perspectives creates complex and meaningful outcomes.

Often, a qualitative approach requires the researcher to spend considerable time in the setting or field simply observing. The researcher takes up a position and takes notes either orally via recording or in written form. Observational studies, such as ethnographies, may require months or even years of immersion in the setting. The detailed notes are then woven into a description of the culture or topic of study.

Historical documents are often consulted during each of the five types of qualitative research. At times, the documents are consulted prior to interviews or observations to help frame the interview questions or observation focus. More commonly, historical documents are reviewed after data collection and analysis to put the findings in a grander context—that is, within the available literature (i.e., the historical documents).[4] Grounding the study outcomes in the available literature in this way brings meaning to the overall topic.

Analyzing Data

Once the data collection is complete, it is time to begin analyzing the data, a process that can vary among the type of qualitative studies. For example, an ethnographic study may include a film of the culture in action. Analysis of the film may involve two or more independent researchers viewing the film and recording their inter- pretations of what they saw. These interpretations may then be compared and combined according to common themes. A phenomenological study, on the other hand, may include four in-depth interviews, each of which may be analyzed and included in the study outcomes independently of the others to provide a full picture of the phenomenon from four perspectives. The following sections describe some basic qualitative data analysis practices.

Reviewing the Data

Completing a general comprehensive review of the collected data is the first step in data analysis because it allows the researcher to look at all of the data at once, usually for the first time. The researcher can then organize the data into whatever system makes sense to begin analysis. The data are commonly put into files and organized.

Reducing the Data

After an initial comprehensive review, true analysis begins. This requires the researcher to read through all of the text and form initial codes. **Coding** is the process by which the researcher identifies themes that occur in the text.[4] Initial coding is performed in each participant transcript or text. From there, thematic or axial coding is performed, which combines the initial codes from each partici- pant's data record into one coding scheme for the full study. Figure 10.6 offers an example of a simple axial coding scheme from a study investigating why athletic training students persist in or leave the profession.[5] The researcher may perform three or more levels of coding until a full description of the study topic is apparent. At times, word counts within codes may be used to express the frequency of the theme in the full data set.

Using Computer Programs for Qualitative Data Analysis

Many software programs are available to help with data reduction via coding. These are collectively called computer-assisted qualitative data analysis programs. They generally operate by loading text from interviews, setting a few sorting parameters, and then hitting the Go button. Skilled users, just as with EBP searches, are more efficient at getting the software to produce the most concise and accurate coding in the shortest time. The output is a coding scheme, which most programs label and color-code based on how often words or phrases occur in the text. The researcher can then sort the output by theme or create new themes to further reduce the data. Researchers report the name, publisher, and edition of the software in the research report.

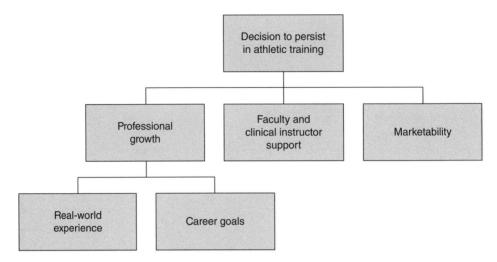

Figure 10.6 Axial coding in a qualitative study.

Reprinted, by permission, from S. Mazerolle et al., 2012, "Undergraduate athletic training students' influences on career decisions after graduation," *Journal of Athletic Training* 47(6): 679-693.

Developing a Theoretical Framework of Study Outcomes

When coding is complete, the researcher forms a theoretical framework of the study outcomes. This is the point at which the researcher identifies a story line that integrates the theme codes into a hypothesis or proposition. Although a qualitative research study does not begin with a hypothesis to be investigated (as quantitative research does), it does begin with a topic that is in need of illumination or understanding. The researcher then collects and analyzes the data and waits for themes to emerge. The result is often a hypothesis related to the topic. A theoretical framework is used to present that hypothesis.

Nesting Outcomes Within the Current Literature

With the study outcomes, themes, and theoretical framework in hand, the researcher needs to situate, or nest, the study within the larger body of research studies on the topic. This process provides a larger context for the study. It also helps to justify the importance of the research study and topic as a whole. This is the final step in the process of data analysis.

Assessing Trustworthiness

As an evidence-based practitioner, you need to ensure that your clinical practice is keeping up with the latest research evidence. This text has helped you to find, understand, and appraise that evidence. To determine whether a research study is of high quality and therefore worthy of your attention, you must consider validity and reliability. Quantitative research provides many statistical measures for validity and reliability. However, qualitative research typically has no statistics

Foundations of Evidence: Strategies to Enhance Validity in Qualitative Research Studies

- Prolonged engagement
- Peer review or an external auditor
- Member checks
- Triangulation
- Negative case analysis
- Clarifying researcher bias

at all. So, how can you determine whether the results of qualitative studies are trustworthy? *Trustworthiness* is the term used by qualitative researchers to denote validity. Other terms you may see in place of *validity* are *credibility, dependability,* and *verification.* The six basic strategies to enhance validity (i.e., ensure trustworthiness) in qualitative research are prolonged engagement, peer review or an external auditor, member checks, triangulation, negative case analysis, and clarifying researcher bias.[1,2,4]

Prolonged engagement refers to a lengthy time spent in the field gathering data. This may include observing, doing interviews and follow-ups, reviewing historical documents, or any combination of these. If you wanted a good understanding of how a field hockey team operates both on and off the field, would you spend a day or a whole season with the team? The qualitative researcher would spend the whole season. The more time the researcher spends in the field, the greater the validity of the study outcomes.

Peer review is a process in which an outside qualitative researcher who is not involved in the study, but is knowledgeable about the topic, provides feedback about the methods, meanings derived from the participants, and interpretations of the authors. Peer reviewers serve as a sort of devil's advocate as they attempt to uncover any errors or holes in the study prior to the writing of the final manuscript. The peer review process may be compared to interrater reliability in quantitative research. Similarly, an **external auditor** may examine both the process (methods, definitions, and interpretations) and the product (the final manuscript) to assess accuracy. External auditors must have no connection whatsoever to the research study. They determine whether the findings, interpretations, and conclusions are supported by the data. This process is also compared to interrater reliability in quantitative research.

Member checks are considered the gold standard of validity in qualitative research. These entail taking the data, analyses, interpretations, and tentative conclusions back to the study participants for their review of the accuracy of the information. This is to ensure that the researcher has captured the information correctly from the participants' perspective. Many qualitative researchers consider member checks to be the most critical technique for establishing validity, trustworthiness, and credibility. Member checks may be done periodically throughout the data collection period or only at the conclusion of the writing process but before publication. Authors should describe how this process was conducted in the research report.

Triangulation is the process in which a researcher uses multiple sources, methods, and investigators to provide collaborative evidence. This is done as data are collected to confirm emerging findings. The theory is that triangulation establishes validity by using the pooled judgments from multiple sources.

Negative case analysis is used when the initial theory of the research is changed as a result of contrary findings as the research moves forward.[4] Essentially, a study begins with the researcher's theory about a topic. If the data collected are contrary to the researcher's theory, the theory is changed to match the findings. This process continues until all data are included.

Researcher bias is presented at the outset of the research and clearly stated in research reports so that readers understand the researcher's position and any biases that may affect the interpretation of the data and thus the conclusions of the study. We all have assumptions or biases when we begin research. Qualitative research embraces this and simply states those biases up front. This is a critical and ethical step in providing validity to a qualitative research study. As you read qualitative studies, look for statements of author bias early in the report so that as you read through the methods, results, discussion, and conclusions, you have a sense of how the stated biases may have influenced the study.

Critical Appraisal of Qualitative Research Studies

To assess the quality of qualitative research studies in athletic training, you need a basic knowledge of this type of research. We offer the following six-step process to guide you through a critical appraisal.[6] During the appraisal, you will refer to the aspects of qualitative research presented earlier in the chapter.

Step 1

The first step is determining whether the study topic is relevant to your clinical question. This is less about judging the quality of the study and more about determining whether you should be spending time completing the rest of the appraisal. Qualitative studies can be lengthy, so be sure your clinical question is directly related to the study you are appraising.

Step 2

Step 2 addresses whether the research approach is appropriate to answer your clinical question. For instance, is the approach used the best choice, given the topic? Doing a biographical study of a person who was a college athlete and an athletic training student to understand the experience of people who fit into these categories through their undergraduate college years might not be the best choice, because many athletic trainers were also college athletes. An ethnographic or grounded theory approach may be more appropriate.

> ## Foundations of Evidence: Six-Step Critical Appraisal Process for Qualitative Research Studies
>
> 1. Is the study topic relevant to your clinical question?
> 2. Was the research approach appropriate for the clinical question?
> 3. Was the sampling method clearly defined and justified?
> 4. Were the data collection methods defined and appropriate?
> 5. What methods were used to analyze the data, and how trustworthy are they?
> 6. Are the conclusions appropriate and accurate, given any stated researcher biases?

Step 3

Step 3 addresses whether the sampling method was clearly defined and justified. This is a difficult area for many athletic trainers because we are taught to use as unbiased a sample as possible in quantitative approaches. However, with qualitative approaches, the sampling is most often very purposeful because we hope to find meaning in the experiences of people who have encountered the topic of investigation. We seek those people; at no time do we attempt to be random in our sampling. What the author of a qualitative study does need to offer is the detailed reasoning behind the sampling method. If this is not clearly defined, then your appraisal of the study may be lower.

You should also assess whether the subjects of the study were representative of the issue being studied. Their characteristics should be well defined. The subjects do not need to have the same characteristics, but they should all belong to the group being studied. Step 3 is also about determining whether appropriate numbers and relationships of subjects were used in the study. For example, in the study to determine the experience of college athletes who were also athletic training students, you would want to interview students from various universities and perhaps even various regions of the country. Subjects from institutions of different sizes may be appropriate to include. People who were not within this demographic but worked closely with these subjects may also be appropriate to include—such as head athletic trainers during the subjects' time at their institutions.

Step 4

In step 4 you determine whether the data collection methods were appropriate. For example, if a study sampled eight people via interview, but the interviews were conducted via phone, without a set script, and only handwritten notes were taken, the quality and accuracy of those notes are questionable. Rather, if those eight people were interviewed in person with a set script of questions and the conversations were recorded for later analysis, those transcriptions would be more reliable. You should be able to identify any bias in the researcher's data collection methods based on the detail in the descriptions of their methods.

Step 5

Step 5 is perhaps the most difficult in the critical appraisal process of qualitative research studies. In this step, you question what methods were used to analyze the data and how trustworthy they are. Reducing the data and developing a theoretical framework of the outcomes with great rigor and quality are daunting tasks. Thus, many qualitative studies fall short in either their data reduction techniques or their trustworthiness. As described early in the chapter, the rigor used by the authors during the assessment of trustworthiness will truly determine the final quality of the study. How did the authors derive themes or concepts from the data? How did they check to be sure those themes were accurate? Did they describe only one aspect of the study topic, or did they present all possible aspects that arose from the data? Did they use more than one method to assess trustworthiness? If so, did they clearly define how those measures of trustworthiness, credibility, or verification were conducted? All of these questions should be answered within the study presentation.

Be cautious in this step about authors who report conducting a specific type of validity measure, such as member checking, but did not fully perform that task. For example, if an author reported performing member checking but did this with only 1 of the 20 participants, this would indicate low validity. Additionally, if that was the only measure of trustworthiness conducted, the validity would score even lower. Most researchers attempt to conduct three types of validity assessments.

Step 6

The last step assesses whether the researchers' conclusions are appropriate and accurate, given any stated biases. Every published qualitative research study should have a clear statement of the researchers' biases, because this helps establish the trustworthiness of the outcomes. Given the stated biases, are the conclusions accurate? Are they overstated? Some authors present their data well but then state conclusions that do not represent those data. This commonly indicates unstated researcher bias. So, be clear about whether the conclusions match the data (i.e., are neither overstated nor understated), given the authors' stated biases.

Time to Practice

Let's put this appraisal process into action. The critical appraisal of evidence on page 151 demonstrates the use of this six-step process. Use this as an example, and then do an EBP search to find another qualitative article that interests you. With that article, perform your own critical appraisal. Practicing appraising qualitative studies will make you more efficient and skilled at interpreting qualitative articles.

Qualitative Research and Athletic Training

Like any profession, athletic training is multifaceted. There are ups and downs, improvements and setbacks, challenges and triumphs for each of us along the way. With the great variation in athletic trainers comes even greater variation in the evidence that informs our clinical practice. No one form or research approach can possibly cover all of the nuances of our profession. Thus, we argue that there

Critical Appraisal of Evidence

In this critical appraisal of evidence, we are evaluating the following qualitative research article:

Mazerolle SM, Pitney WA, Goodman A. Retention factors
for head athletic trainers in the NCAA Division I collegiate setting.
IJATT. 2012; 18 (4): 10-13.

Study Overview

This grounded theory study investigated factors that influenced the retention of head athletic trainers (ATs) at NCAA Division I institutions.

Critical Appraisal

1. *Is the study topic relevant to my clinical question?* Yes.

2. *Was the research approach appropriate for the clinical question?* Yes, using grounded theory to link the interview results via coding was appropriate.

3. *Was the sampling method clearly defined and justified?* The researchers solicited participants using purposeful sampling through e-mails sent to 20 head ATs at NCAA Division I institutions. Eighteen of the 20 people contacted agreed to participate. This was appropriate sampling and clearly defined.

4. *Were the data collection methods defined and appropriate?* The data collection method of an online survey was defined. However, this was not an appropriate method of gathering data. Online surveys should not be used in place of live interviews. The lack of interviewer–interviewee interaction with online surveys dramatically limits the quality and richness of the data received.

5. *What methods were used to analyze the data, and how trustworthy are they?* The researchers proposed that their "inductive analysis process" was comparable to open coding, which is questionable. They also stated that they took "field notes in the margins of the transcripts." This is questionable because field notes require the researcher to be in the field. What exactly this means is unclear. Thus, the authors' coding lacked rigor. They established trustworthiness, or credibility, by employing member checks (though of two "supervisors" rather than participants), peer review (by one of the authors), and a minimal form of triangulation (comparing two investigators' findings). Thus, the overall appraisal of data analysis and trustworthiness is fair at best.

6. *Were the conclusions made by the researchers appropriate and accurate, given any stated researcher biases?* No researcher biases were stated at any point throughout the article. Further, the report included no negative comments from the participants. Thus, the picture provided is very limited and appears one-sided. It is difficult to determine whether the conclusions are accurate.

is no place for either a strictly quantitative or a strictly qualitative approach to inform the profession. Rather, each researcher must determine which approach best suits the clinical question. Many researchers prefer to conduct research within one approach, which is acceptable as long as the questions to be investigated are fitting for that approach.

Pure Qualitative Approach

Qualitative research provides rich descriptions of the human experience within certain contexts. Many areas of athletic training include contexts that defy explanation by numbers or statistics—particularly those that deal with human emotions. Examples include what clinical preceptors believe about the best way to help students learn, how students feel about mentorship, and how athletes manage their emotions about being injured. None of those areas could be well defined by statistics. However, performing several in-depth interviews or spending six months in the field immersed in that context would provide rich descriptions of what those experiences mean to the subjects, which can inform our clinical practice. Consider that many qualitative studies performed in the 1990s and early 2000s resulted in an increased emphasis on the psychosocial aspects of injured athletes in AT education.

Pure Quantitative Approach

As you have seen through a majority of this text, there is clearly a place and time for purely quantitative approaches in athletic training. When determining optimal modality settings for specific injuries, for example, there is less interest in the subjects' experience of that modality and more interest in the amount of tissue temperature change to promote healing. The majority of evidence in most health care professions comes from the quantitative approach. However, because health care involves humans, qualitative studies are needed for understanding the human experience.

Mixed-Methods Approach

Many studies in athletic training use what is called a **mixed-methods approach**, an approach that uses both quantitative and qualitative methods. This approach is ideal in some situations. For example, currently in athletic training and beyond, there is a great interest in concussion research. Concussions are inherently difficult to study because we struggle to quantify the severity and breadth of each occurrence. Athletes experience concussions in very different ways, which cannot yet be explained with imaging techniques. We have to rely mostly on self-reports of symptoms and computerized tests that measure aspects such as reaction time, cognition, and balance, which athletes can control to some extent. Thus, many current research projects attempt to decrease the chance that athletes might be able to "cheat the test." Some studies include the qualitative process of interviewing athletes about why this culture of cheating the test exists. Given the clear evidence that permanent and debilitating brain damage can occur with repetitive concussions, why do many athletes persist in hiding them? This is an area that lends itself well to a mixed-methods approach.

A complicating factor with the mixed-methods approach is that some researchers are not well versed in qualitative methods. Often, the qualitative piece is poorly designed and lacks rigor, as revealed in the analysis section. Simply asking participants to fill in a comment box on a survey does not represent qualitative research. So, as an evidence-based clinician, use caution when appraising these types of studies.

Summary

This chapter reviewed the basic concepts of qualitative research. The five types of qualitative research (ethnography, phenomenology, grounded theory, case study, and biography) were presented and defined. Examples of how each type of study may be used in athletic training were provided. This was followed by descriptions of how qualitative study sampling and data collection are typically conducted. The more complicated processes of data analysis and assessing trustworthiness (validity and reliability) were presented in detail. A six-step critical appraisal of qualitative research process was provided along with an application exercise for practicing a critical appraisal. A discussion of how qualitative research should be used in athletic training concluded the chapter.

References

1. Creswell JW. *Qualitative inquiry and research design: Choosing among five traditions.* Thousand Oaks, CA: Sage; 1998: 402.

2. Merriam S. *Qualitative research and case study applications in education.* San Francisco: Jossey-Bass; Wiley; 2001.

3. Webber M. *Dropping the bucket and sponge: A history of early athletic training 1881-1947.* Prescott, AZ: Athletic Training History; 2013.

4. Giacomini MK, Cook CD. Users' guides to the medical literature: XXIII. Qualitative research in health care A. Are the results of the study valid? Evidence-based medicine working group. *JAMA.* 2000; 284: 357-362.

5. Mazerolle S, Gavin K, Pitney W, Casa D, Burton L. Undergraduate athletic training students' influences on career decisions after graduation. *J Athl Train.* 2012; 47 (6): 679-692.

6. Giacomini MK, Cook CD. Users' guides to the medical literature: XXIII. Qualitative research in health care B. What are the results and how do they help me care for my patients? Evidence-based medicine working group. *JAMA.* 2000; 284: 478-483.

CHAPTER 11

Research Ethics

Objectives

After reading this chapter, you will be able to do the following:

- Explain why researchers need to be ethical.
- Describe the process of informed consent and its purpose.
- Understand the purpose of IRBs and their function.
- Understand the negative impact of unethical research and reporting.

Asking for forgiveness instead of permission regarding research and publications is never acceptable. All research should be beyond reproach. Most researchers want to find answers to questions or solve new problems because they genuinely care about people. However, they also face external pressure in their academic settings to "publish or perish." The pressure to publish causes some researchers to fudge data, adjust the reporting of their statistics, or not report failures. Taking shortcuts that might not be illegal to speed up the process or save money when funds are short is unethical behavior that can be tempting. However, for the profession of athletic training to move forward, the members of the National Athletic Trainers' Association (NATA) and the readers of athletic training research must be able to trust what we publish and that we have protected the participants in our studies.

Ethical Roadblocks

Researchers who follow solid ethical codes, work hard, and treat their subjects fairly and honestly may reap few rewards. This is especially true if they lack funds, resources, or lab space; have difficulty recruiting participants; and fail to have their research published. Researchers in this position often feel like failures and receive no acknowledgments from their institutions. Many lose their jobs. When facing this possibility, some may ask themselves, What is the harm in fudging data? What is so wrong about inflating the impact of my results if it helps me get published and retain my job? Researchers internalize these cognitive struggles based on their own beliefs and interactions with other scientists, their professional training, and the emphasis the profession places on ethical behavior.[1]

The profession of athletic training, the *Journal of Athletic Training*, other allied health care providers, and companies that fund research oppose scientific misconduct. **Scientific misconduct** is when researchers fail to report their methods or results accurately. A researcher may complete a study but misrepresent it in the reporting. Some researchers have actually not conducted any research and then fabricated entire studies along with fake participants, fake methods, and fake data yielding spurious results and conclusions. Although rare, when such **research fraud** is discovered, it is punished severely.[1] **Plagiarism,** the copying of another person's work without providing credit to that person, is another act that is always unethical but may not be illegal (e.g., when the copied work is not explicitly protected by a contract, confidentiality agreement, or copyright).

Principles of Ethics

Ethics in research addresses issues beyond how the publish-or-perish world affects the researcher. The increased cultural awareness of the need for evidence-based practice and research has increased the need for research with human subjects. With this comes a responsibility to protect human subjects from actions that negatively affect their dignity or psychological or physical well-being.[2] To this end, universities and health care organizations such as hospitals and government agencies now require researchers to complete ethics training and to submit research proposals to an institutional review board (IRB) prior to embarking on studies involving humans or animals. The Collaborative Institutional Training Initiative (CITI) at the University of Miami is an online resource used by institutions to ensure that researchers are familiar with ethical guidelines. For more information about CITI, or to complete training modules, visit www.citiprogram.org.

Additional ethical issues are the simultaneous submission of manuscripts to multiple journals, duplicate or redundant publications, and ghost authorship. The *Journal of Athletic Training*'s (*JAT*'s) "Authors' Guide" has a form authors sign stating that their work has been solely submitted to the *JAT* and is not under other review (the form is available at www.journalofathletictraining.org). Multiple submissions waste reviewers' time and may result in duplicate publications (the same article published in two publications without reference to each other).

The *JAT*'s "Authors' Guide" also requests that authors declare that they have put a significant amount of effort into the manuscript and that each contributor is identified, including those involved in concept development, design, and data collection; drafting and revising the article; and approving the final version. It further states that any of these tasks alone, securing the general funding for a project, and supervising the project do not constitute authorship. This wording leaves open the possibility of interpretations that can lead to ghost authorship.

According to the International Committee of Medical Journal Editors (ICMJE) and the Council of Scientific Editors (CSE), ghost authorship is the suppression of the name of a person who made a significant contribution to a portion or all of a study.[3] This can occur when senior researchers or professors leave off the names of junior colleagues or students. A troublesome practice is the completing of clinical studies by drug companies that, to avoid the appearance of financial conflict or bias, hire scientific writers to submit their articles. This significantly undercuts the trust readers place in authors.

Foundations of Evidence: Six Principles of Ethics

1. Beneficence: Demonstrate that the project will benefit the participants or population.
2. Nonmaleficence: Do no harm.
3. Fidelity: Never put the research above the participants' welfare.
4. Justice: Treat all participants equally and fairly.
5. Veracity: Never deceive participants.
6. Confidentiality: Ensure that participants are unidentifiable.

Following are six ethical principles to consider when designing a research study.[2]

1. **Beneficence.** Beneficence states that the project should have an intended benefit for the participants or the greater population. A study should not be conducted merely for the sake of doing research; clear goals should be detailed.

2. **Nonmaleficence.** In keeping with the spirit of the Hippocratic Oath, which says "Do no harm," the goal of nonmaleficence is to protect participants from long-term or short-term physical or emotional pain or danger.

3. **Fidelity.** Fidelity is faithfulness to people or beliefs. As a principle of ethics, it refers to participants' trust that the researcher will not harm them.

4. **Justice.** Justice obliges a researcher to treat all participants equally and fairly. Although important, this principle challenges the typical research design in which one group is treated and another group is not. In these types of studies, researchers should inform participants that one group will be treated and the other will be provided a placebo or a typically accepted treatment. If the researcher discovers that a participant in the placebo group has a condition that is worsening and it can be treatable with other measures, he should withdraw that participant and provide her with the best treatment currently available.

5. **Veracity.** Veracity refers to truthfulness; participants should not be deceived at any time. They should be made aware of the expected outcomes, the aims of the study, and any potential side effects of treatments or interventions.

6. **Confidentiality.** Confidentiality requires that participants not be identified to anyone outside of the research team. When data are disseminated, all names or personally identifiable information about participants should be removed. Data that are stored should be coded to prevent accidental discovery of the participants' health information by people outside the research team.

History of Ethics

After World War II, policies were formed to prevent doctors from carrying out experiments on prisoners without their consent. The Nuremberg Code, written for use in military tribunals aimed at bringing doctors to trial, asserted that human subjects must voluntarily consent to be subjects. However, the unethical treatment of human subjects continued after the Nuremberg Code was established. The most notable case was the Tuskegee Study, conducted by the U.S. government. Poor African-American men with syphilis were allowed to suffer so the researchers could watch the disease progression even though a cure had been found. The Declaration of Helsinki went further than the Nuremberg Code by declaring not only that participants had to volunteer but also that the purpose of research involving human subjects must be to improve diagnostic, therapeutic, or prophylactic procedures and to increase our understanding of disease causes and progressions. In 1966, the U.S. National Institutes of Health (NIH) adopted these policies to safeguard human subjects; they became regulations in 1974 when the IRB process was established. Between 1974 and 1978, the National Commission for the Protection of Human Subjects in Biomedical and Behavioral Research in the United States defined the principles of ethical research to protect human subjects. The resulting outcome is referred to as the Belmont Report.[4]

Nuremberg Code

1. The voluntary consent of the human subject is absolutely essential.

   This means that the person involved should have legal capacity to give consent; should be so situated as to be able to exercise free power of choice, without the intervention of any element of force, fraud, deceit, duress, over-reaching, or other ulterior form of constraint or coercion; and should have sufficient knowledge and comprehension of the elements of the subject matter involved, as to enable him to make an understanding and enlightened decision. This latter element requires that, before the acceptance of an affirmative decision by the experimental subject, there should be made known to him the nature, duration, and purpose of the experiment; the method and means by which it is to be conducted; all inconveniences and hazards reasonably to be expected; and the effects upon his health or person, which may possibly come from his participation in the experiment.

   The duty and responsibility for ascertaining the quality of the consent rests upon each individual who initiates, directs or engages in the experiment. It is a personal duty and responsibility which may not be delegated to another with impunity.

2. The experiment should be such as to yield fruitful results for the good of society, unprocurable by other methods or means of study, and not random and unnecessary in nature.

3. The experiment should be so designed and based on the results of animal experimentation and a knowledge of the natural history of the disease or other problem under study, that the anticipated results will justify the performance of the experiment.

4. The experiment should be so conducted as to avoid all unnecessary physical and mental suffering and injury.

5. No experiment should be conducted, where there is an *apriori* reason to believe that death or disabling injury will occur; except, perhaps, in those experiments where the experimental physicians also serve as subjects.

6. The degree of risk to be taken should never exceed that determined by the humanitarian importance of the problem to be solved by the experiment.

7. Proper preparations should be made and adequate facilities provided to protect the experimental subject against even remote possibilities of injury, disability, or death.

8. The experiment should be conducted only by scientifically qualified persons. The highest degree of skill and care should be required through all stages of the experiment of those who conduct or engage in the experiment.

9. During the course of the experiment, the human subject should be at liberty to bring the experiment to an end, if he has reached the physical or mental state, where continuation of the experiment seemed to him to be impossible.

10. During the course of the experiment, the scientist in charge must be prepared to terminate the experiment at any stage, if he has probable cause to believe, in the exercise of the good faith, superior skill and careful judgement required of him, that a continuation of the experiment is likely to result in injury, disability, or death to the experimental subject.

Reprinted from *Trials of war criminals before the Nuremberg Military Tribunals under control council law no. 10*, Vol. 2, 1949 (Washington, D.C.: U.S. Government Printing Office), 181-182.

Although reviewing the entire Belmont Report is informative, it can be summarized in four key points:

1. Research designs should be valid to increase the likelihood of meaningful results.

2. The researcher should be competent and proficient in the skills required to complete the research procedures.

3. To minimize risk and ensure benefits, researchers should assess the methods from all perspectives and ensure that subjects selected for the study represent the benefiting population.

4. The subjects must give voluntary consent and be capable of doing so. Researchers are responsible for any harm experienced by the subjects.[5]

The Belmont Report is available in its entirety at www.hhs.gov/ohrp/human-subjects/guidance/belmont.html. The 18th World Medical Association (WMA) general assembly adopted the Declaration of Helsinki in June 1964. It was established as a statement of ethical principles that all medical researchers involving human subjects, including human material, should abide by. It is to be understood and followed as a complete set of directions and not broken down into separate paragraphs for micro-interpretation. To view the Declaration of Helsinki in its entirely, go to this site: http://science.education.nih.gov/supplements/nih9/bioethics/guide/teacher/Mod5_Helsinki.pdf.

Institutional Review Board (IRB) Process

A primary interest of every researcher in the health and human sciences must be the protection of participants. The institutional review board (IRB) at a researcher's selected institution is tasked with ensuring that no harm comes to subjects of research studies. The IRB requires that participants receive informed consent, which means that they are made aware of their rights. The informed consent documents state that participants knowingly, willingly, and rationally take part in the research free from any coercion. If the research involves minors, the consent must come from parents or guardians, but the children also have to consent to participate. If participants are too young to understand, elderly, confused, or psychiatrically disturbed, the informed consent process is more difficult; in this case, the IRB reviews the details of the research plan to ensure subject protection.[2]

Research participants must be made aware of their right to discontinue participation in a study at any time, regardless of the impact it may have on the study or the researcher. The researcher cannot coerce or refuse participants the right to future participation or treatment as a result of dropping out of the study.

When appraising research, it is prudent to pay attention to the reporting of the research. A researcher should always state that IRB approval was gained prior to conducting any research or data collection. If such a statement is not included, the study may lack validity or measures to protect subjects, and using the information for clinical decisions is thus problematic.

Trustworthiness and Conflicts

Researchers face other ethical issues in addition to the welfare of their participants. Conflicts of interest include the influence of corporate sponsors as well as the researcher's financial interest in the products used in the study. They also include personal relationships between authors and their sponsors or journal editorial boards. Additional ethical issues are misinterpretations of data and authorship rights when multiple researchers are involved in a study. Journal reviewers may also more favorably review studies that support an effective or new treatment. Finally, an author can simply create results or ignore the actual outcomes in favor of something else.

Conflicts of interest are common and should be part of every article appraisal. Authors often declare that a company funded the research they conducted. This is often a prerequisite of receiving funds. However, the funds should not be dependent on the outcomes reported or limited to methods that will enhance the company funding the research. It is perfectly acceptable for a company to research its product to test it for efficacy. However, those are internal studies, not studies to educate the public; their goal is to enhance the market share of a company.

Consider a researcher who has created a new sport drink that is purported to reduce dehydration and cramping. The researcher needs to secure funding from an independent source such as the NIH to test this new product. It is unlikely that an established sport drink company would want to underwrite a project that may introduce a competitor to the marketplace. On a certain level, this makes sense; however, if companies purport that they truly want to put the health of athletes first and profits second, then maybe they should support such research.

Now consider research submitted for publication that was funded by an established supplier of sports medicine materials purchased by many athletic trainers. If a reviewer for a journal is assessing the article, stripped of the author's name but not of a statement that the project was funded by a well-known and respected supplier that also supports the same journal, is that reviewer able to remain unbiased? Either way, it is an ethical issue that the reviewer will have to consider. Editorial staffs in this type of situation should separate the author name and funding source from the body of the article submission to prevent the potential appearance of unethical influences by the reviewers. Authors should also report any family relation they have with funding agencies or publication companies. It would be unethical to have a company employee decide on the funding of a family member's project. Publications and researchers should always be beyond reproach.

Researchers also need to ensure the adequate and appropriate reporting of their results. If you recall, when initiating a study, the authors must state that they have the technical ability to complete the study. This includes the appropriate and correct interpretation of statistical data and reporting. Literature reviews that solely review study statistics sometimes find errors that result in redactions of articles and resubmissions. Some errors are so gross or the authors so negligent that the authors' works are banned from future publication in peer-reviewed journals.

Issues of authorship have certainly torn apart research teams and ruined the prospect of future collaborative efforts. Typically, the person who develops the idea or carries out the largest portion of the research is the primary author. Although this seems cut and dried, what if an author conceives an idea for a project but less than halfway through leaves the remainder of the data collection and writing to the collaborative research team? Who gets authorship, and in what order are the authors listed? It is a good practice to discuss the contributions of each author before starting a research project and to have a plan for contingencies.

To consider another ethical issue, let's assume that a researcher sets out to answer a clinical question. Unknown to the researcher, four other researchers have the same question and a similar approach to answering it. All have submitted their research for publication in their professional journal, and all have been denied. They were denied not because of poor methods, faulty data, or a failure to protect subjects; rather, the publication stated that the outcomes do not contribute to the advancement of the profession or the results cannot be applied to a relevant population. The problem here is not a violation of ethics on the part of the authors but a question of the goal of the journal. The journal's goal should be to disseminate information from research studies that are well thought out and completed diligently. This should include reporting failures if the methods used were correct. This informs others that a particular approach to a relevant clinical question might not work. Thus, other researchers won't unknowingly replicate a failed research project and waste time and resources.

Let's look at a current event that will likely end up in court. The National Strength and Conditioning Association's (NSCA's) premier publication, the *Journal of Strength and Conditioning Research,* published an article that underwent a rigorous peer review, as do all submitted articles, and was accepted for publication. The content of the article was not favorably received by CrossFit, Inc. CrossFit would like the article withdrawn, and the NSCA at present has not agreed to do so. The NSCA has stated that the article was reviewed and accepted for publication and that it will stand behind the author. This is an important stance for the NSCA to take because if every published article that called current practices into question was retracted as a result of pressure from an organization, we would not be undertaking evidenced-based practice. However, what if the author of any of these articles intentionally falsified the outcomes and committed an ethical error? What is the acceptable outcome, and who is ultimately responsible? These are tough questions. What if the author did not intentionally commit an ethical violation but by an act of omission failed to correctly interpret the data? How should this be handled? Ultimately, these are issues that professionals have to review and consider.

Critical Appraisal of Evidence

To understand why some authors are less than transparent in their research or exercise some freedoms in research, we need to look at certain academic environments. Researchers often believe that if they fail to produce a certain number of publications, they will lose their jobs. This is supported by certain tenure and promotion standards that identify a minimum number of publications expected. Add to that a recent trend at many journals of publishing only articles that have positive outcomes, and you can see why researchers might be biased or fish for numbers to support their hypotheses.

To retain high ethical standards, many journals now have a process of preregistration of studies to be published. The researcher submits the literature review, methods, purpose, and intended statistics to address the research question before conducting the study. If the review committee accepts the presubmission, it guarantees publication regardless of whether the outcome is positive or negative. The researcher must only follow the proposal. For more information regarding the preregistration process, visit http://clinicaltrials.gov or http://centerforopenscience.org.

Summary

The researcher has the ultimate responsibility of protecting study participants. Study participants must understand the risks, participate voluntarily, and be cognitively capable of providing consent. Researchers must submit their research plans to outside reviewers to ensure the safety of participants. It is never acceptable to start a study with human subjects without prior approval and review from the appropriate IRB or other governing agency. In addition to protecting the participants, the researcher must be capable of completing all the tasks involved with the study or have amassed a team to ensure full completion and interpretation of the outcomes. Researchers must also report any potential conflicts of interest so that reviewers and readers can weigh the clinical significance of the study. The ultimate goal of research and publications is to provide meaningful and trustworthy information.

References

1. Neuman L. *Social research methods; qualitative and quantitative approaches*. 4th ed. Needham Heights, MA: Allyn & Bacon; 2000.

2. Hicks C. *Research methods for clinical therapists, applied project design and analysis*. 5th ed. New York: Churchill Livingstone; 2009.

3. Bavdekar S. Authorship issues. *Lung India*. 2012; 29 (1): 76-80.

4. Ingersoll C. *Research in athletic training*. Thorofare, NJ: Slack; 2001.

5. Gliner J, Morgan G. *Research methods in applied settings: An integrated approach to design and analysis*. Mahwah, NJ: Erlbaum; 2000: 465.

Glossary

accuracy—Refers to a precise measure; it says that the value is true.

altruism—The belief in the value of acting for others' good; selflessness.

apps—Electronic applications for use with mobile devices.

a priori—An analysis determining the needed p value to signify significance prior to collecting data.

arithmetic mean—The average of all scores; normally denoted in articles by the symbol $\bar{x}$.

biography—The study of one person's experiences as told to a researcher in person or via historical documents.

Boolean search—A search technique that uses the operator words *AND, OR*, and *NOT* to combine search terms to gain detailed search results.

case control studies—Retrospective reviews of portions of a population who present with an injury or illness after it occurs and comparing those to others who do not present with the condition and looking for possible contributory factors.

case studies—In qualitative research, studies that investigate a confined topic with a focus on either the individual case or an issue that is illustrated by the case.

clinical expertise—The culmination of the athletic trainer's experience treating and providing care to athletes.

clinical meaningfulness—An outcome measure's ability to provide measures of change in the athlete's condition that are valuable to the athlete and the clinician.

clinical practice guidelines (CPGs)—Guidelines that incorporate evidence from research, clinical expertise, and athletes' perspectives.

clinical research—A scientific and systematic process that generates evidence through hypothesis testing and sound methodology.

coding—A process by which the researcher identifies themes that occur in the text.

Cohen's kappa—A statistic reported as κ that has values between 0 and 1. Values closer to 1 indicate greater agreement between raters. Kappa is a measure of true agreement beyond what would occur by chance alone.

cohort study—A study that follows a similar group of people likely to develop a condition in the future to establish the percentage of people who actually develop the condition after an extended time.

confidence interval—An estimate of the chance variation expected with similar studies.

content validity—A form of validity determined when a group of experts reviews the instrument, often a questionnaire or survey, and arrives at a consensus that the instrument covers aspects of the concept it is intended to measure.

correlation—A statistical relationship between two variables.

criterion validity—The ability of an instrument or assessment to correlate with an established assessment.

critically appraised topic (CAT)—A one-page summary of the literature appraisal and clinical relevance of a clinical topic. Commonly, few basic research articles are used to inform the CAT summary.

cross-sectional study—A study that provides data about the prevalence of a condition across a population of interest at one point in time.

database—An online collection of research articles.

dependent variable—A variable of interest that is affected by other variables in a study.

diagnostic accuracy—A summary of measures such as sensitivity and specificity of various tests, allowing a clinician to arrive at a conclusion.

disablement theory—A theory that states that acute and chronic injury or illness affects the body's systems—physical and mental—thereby affecting activities of daily living. The athletic trainer must consider this to treat the athlete as a whole person.

effect size—A value that reflects the magnitude of the treatment effect or the strength of the relationship between two variables.

eligibility criteria—A set of delimiters that detail who can be included in a study.

ethnography—The study of an intact cultural or social group via observations and a prolonged time spent in the field.

evidence—Research study outcomes that are published.

evidence-based practice (EBP)—A systematic method of reviewing the best evidence, combining it with the art of athletic training or the athletic trainer's clinical expertise, and making informed choices to treat the athlete.

external auditor—A person who examines both the process of a quantitative study (methods, definitions, and interpretations) and its product (the final manuscript) to assess accuracy. The auditor must have no connections whatsoever to the research study.

face validity—A form of validity that establishes only that the instrument seems to measure what it is intended to measure.

false negative—When a test incorrectly identifies a condition or illness as not present when it is present.

false positive—When a test indicates the presence of a condition that in reality does not exist.

filtered information—Studies that have been evaluated along with multiple similar studies by someone other than the researcher and then combined with those studies to form a comprehensive review of outcomes for a particular topic.

generalizability—The extent to which the results of a study can be applied to a different population.

global rating of change (GRC)—Athlete-rated change as an outcome measure to determine the efficacy of a rehabilitation plan, progression, or treatment.

gold standard—A test, technique, or measure that is most commonly used across clinicians within a profession, such as clinical special tests for orthopedic conditions. A diagnostic test used as a benchmark to compare other tests to, which may not be perfect but is acceptable.

grounded theory—A type of qualitative study that requires the researcher to generate a theory that explains some action, interaction, or process.

health-related quality of life—Physical and mental health perceptions (health risks and conditions, functional status, social support, and socioeconomic status) that affect the outcome of injury rehabilitation.

HIPAA—Health Insurance Portability and Accountability Act.

incidental sampling—A sample of convenience based on access.

independent variable—A variable not affected by the study or other variables being measured.

internal reliability—A form or reliability that considers whether similar questions on the same instrument are answered similarly by a participant.

interrater reliability—Agreement between clinicians when they perform independent assessments of a condition.

interval—The level of quantitative data that provides consistent differences between intervals.

intrarater reliability—The reproducibility of a clinical measure when performed by the same clinician on more than one occasion on the same athlete.

known-groups validity— The ability of an assessment to differentiate correctly between groups of people with a condition and groups of people without it.

likelihood ratio—A ratio that uses the sensitivity and specificity of a test to help clinicians determine decisions.

Likert scale—A rating scale named for Rensis Likert, an educator and organizational psychologist, that is used to assess preferences between two polar opposites.

mean—See arithmetic mean.

measures of central tendency—Measures that revolve around the mean, median, and mode and cluster around the center of the normal distribution.

median score—The score that falls in the middle of a distribution.

member check—The process of taking the data, analyses, interpretations, and tentative conclusions of a study back to the participants for their review of the accuracy of the information.

MeSH search—A search technique that uses medical subject heading terms that are chosen from a preset list in some medical databases. The lists start general and become more specific as you choose terms in a stepwise method.

meta-analysis—A scientific method of statistical combination of several research study outcomes or results to produce an estimate of the effect of an intervention.

metasearch engine—A search engine that presents only meta-analyses consolidated from other search engines.

minimal clinically important difference (MCID)—An athlete-derived score that reflects changes in injury status as a result of a clinical intervention that are meaningful for the athlete.

minimal detectable change (MDC)—The amount of change needed to exceed a natural variation and represent true change in the athlete's injury recovery.

mixed-methods approach—A research approach that uses both quantitative and qualitative methods.

mode—The most commonly occurring value in a distribution of numeric data.

My NCBI—A tool through PubMed that allows you to receive alerts when new research articles on topics of interest are published.

negative case analysis—Changing the initial theory of the research as a result of contrary findings as the research moves forward.

negative correlation—The relationship between two constructs in which one construct score increases as the other decreases.

negative predictive value—The percentage of people who test negative for a condition as identified by the gold standard assessment for that condition.

nominal—The level of quantitative data that provides names for variables (e.g., group A).

nomogram—A device for calculating the posttest probability of a condition based on pretest suspicion and the likelihood ratio of the assessment used in a clinical evaluation.

nonparametric—A category of data that are not normally distributed.

ordinal—The level of quantitative data that provides names or categories for variables that are in order, or ranked.

outcome measure—Any characteristic measured to assess how an athlete is progressing or feeling in the moment.

parametric—A category of data that fall in a normal distribution that allows researchers to draw conclusions mathematically.

patient values—The preconceived ideas and beliefs each athlete brings to a clinical setting.

peer review—A process in which an outside qualitative researcher who is not involved in the study, but is knowledgeable about the topic, provides feedback about the methods, definitions, and interpretations of the study author.

phenomenological studies—Qualitative studies that describe the meaning people ascribe to a certain phenomenon, topic, or concept.

PICO—An acronym for patient or problem, intervention, comparison, outcome.

plagiarism—The copying of another person's work without providing credit to that person.

podcasts—Video or audio electronic media used to disseminate information.

positive correlation—The relationship between two constructs in which one construct score increases as the other increases.

positive predictive value—The percentage of people who test positive for a condition as identified by the gold standard assessment for that condition.

practice effect—Learning how to perform better on a test simply by taking the test.

preappraised resources—Databases that contain only articles that have been critically appraised for quality.

predictive validity—The ability of an assessment to predict an event or outcome.

prevalence—How often an event or condition occurs in a population.

prognostic research—Research focused on foreseeing, or predicting, conditions or outcomes.

prolonged engagement—A lengthy time spent in the field gathering data.

prospective study—A study that follows a group of similar people (e.g., athletes) over a period of time to determine whether certain factors or conditions affect injury prevalence.

psychometric properties—The intrinsic properties of an outcome measure.

pull technology—Databases and search engines that you enter to pull information out to address your clinical question.

purposeful sampling—The process by which the qualitative researcher chooses participants based on their exposure to or experience with the research topic.

push technology—Electronic programs that automatically push information to your computer, e-mail inbox, smartphone, or a combination of these.

qualitative research—Research used to provide a deeper understanding of events or conditions that a person, a group, or an entire culture has experienced.

quantifiable—Able to be measured in exact values and expressed as a number; should be reproducible between assessors.

quantitative research—Research that uses numbers and mathematical equations to test hypotheses in an unbiased manner.

quasi-experimental study—A study that is set up like an experimental design but lacks random assignment, which complicates the interpretation of outcomes based on treatments or grouping.

randomization—A characteristic that helps to determine whether something truly made an impact or whether it might have occurred by chance alone or as a result of a preconceived bias.

randomized controlled trial (RCT)—A trial that begins with a similar group of participants representative of a population of interest. Participants are randomly assigned to either a control group receiving no treatment (or a sham group receiving a placebo) or a treatment (intervention) group.

ratio—The level of quantitative data that has a true zero value.

receiver operating characteristic (ROC) curves—A graphic plot of the sensitivity and specificity values generated by cut points. The cut points determine the number of true positives, true negatives, false positives, and false negatives to minimize errors in clinical diagnoses.

referenced standard—A standard that serves as an acceptable comparison for other measures of interest.

regression—A statistical process in which relationships between variables are compared to predict the value of another outcome variable.

reliability—The ability of an instrument, tool, or person to produce consistent results when measuring the same subject again and again.

representative sample—A subset of a population that would accurately reflect the characteristics of the population.

research fraud—The fabrication of a report or a study that never occurred.

researcher bias—Any bias on the part of researchers, which should be presented at the outset of the research and clearly stated in research reports.

retrospective study—A historical review of an athlete's or population's medical history to identify risk factors of certain conditions.

RSS feed (Really Simple Syndication)—A tool available through some e-mail servers, organizations, or journals that allows you to receive alerts when new research articles on topics of interest are published.

scientific misconduct—When researchers fail to report their methods or results accurately.

search engine—A tool used for searching one or more databases.

sensitivity—The expression of how accurately an assessment can identify a problem or illness.

specificity—The expression of how accurately an assessment can identify the absence of a problem or illness.

stratified sampling—Sampling from each subgroup in a population.

subjective—Lacking exactly reproducible numeric values and influenced by people's opinions; may vary from person to person.

systematic review (SR)—A scientific tool that can be used to appraise, summarize, and communicate the results and implications of otherwise unmanageable quantities of research. These reviews go through a rigorous process of appraisal and synthesis.

systemic sampling—Sampling based on an interval or systematic process.

test–retest reliability—The ability of an instrument or assessment to produce similar outcomes in the same group of people on multiple occasions in an amount of time that would not lead to a change in the measurement of interest.

time series—A collection of quantitative observations that are evenly spaced in time and measured successively.

triangulation—The process in which a researcher uses multiple sources and methods to gather collaborative evidence.

true experimental design—Studies that use random assignment and a control group; they control the variables to be studied.

true negative—When a test correctly identifies the absence of a condition or illness.

true positive—When a test correctly identifies the presence of a condition or illness.

trustworthiness—A term used by qualitative researchers to denote validity.

unfiltered information—Information from research studies whose methods are not evaluated piece by piece in combination with other studies.

validity—The extent to which an instrument, tool, observation, or full study measures what it is intended to measure and the extent to which that measurement is relevant.

vet—To scrutinize.

Index

Note: Page numbers followed by an italicized *f* or *t* refer to the figure or table on that page, respectively.

About the Authors

Scot Raab, PhD, AT, LAT, is an assistant professor in the athletic training education program at Northern Arizona University in Flagstaff. Raab earned his PhD in teaching and administration and has more than 20 years of experience in clinical practice, higher education instruction, and methodological review to contribute to education in evidence-based practice. He teaches several research courses and mentors undergraduate and graduate students in research projects.

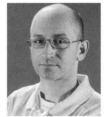

Courtesy of Scot Raab

Debbie I. Craig, PhD, AT, LAT, is the director of the athletic training education program in the department of physical therapy and athletic training and a professor at Northern Arizona University in Flagstaff. With more than a decade of clinical practice in athletic training and a PhD in educational leadership, Craig is an authority in evidence-based practice and research protocols. She teaches EBP to graduate students and is a member of the National Athletic Trainers' Association.

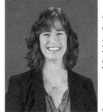

Courtesy of Debbie Craig

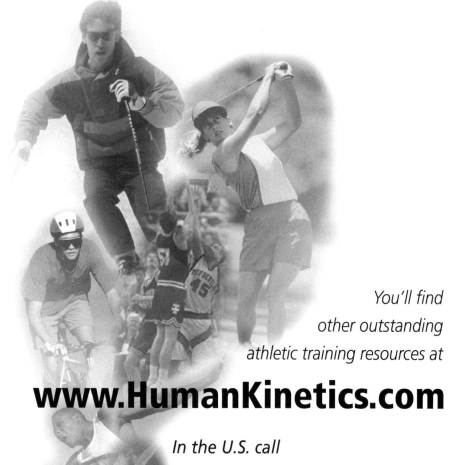